the oneplan

A Week-by-Week Guide

to

RESTORING YOUR NATURAL HEALTH and HAPPINESS

YOGI CAMERON
ALBORZIAN

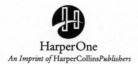

HarperOne
An Imprint of HarperCollinsPublishers

HarperOne

HarperCollins books may be purchased for educational, business, or sales promotional use. For information please email the Special Markets Department at SPsales@harpercollins.com.

HarperCollins website: http://www.harpercollins.com

HarperCollins®, 📖®, and HarperOne™
are trademarks of HarperCollins Publishers

FIRST EDITION

Library of Congress Cataloging-in-Publication Data is available upon request.

ISBN 978–0–06–220583–4

13 14 15 16 17   RRD(H)   10 9 8 7 6 5 4 3 2 1

contents

the
oneplan

introduction

I FIRST MET MARIA MENOUNOS IN 2009, WHEN SHE DID A STORY ON MY WORK with Ayurveda and Yoga for the *Today* show. We became good friends, but we never talked in greater detail about my work on the Yogic path. That is, until about a year later.

At the end of 2010, Maria was suffering from a rash that consumed her entire body. Though this would be bad in any situation, she was slated to cover the Emmy Awards for *Access Hollywood,* and the dress she was planning to wear would leave much of her skin exposed. And while it was unsightly, more than anything she was in pain. The heat of the season only made matters worse. It was only a week and a half until the awards show. None of the medicines she had been prescribed were helping. When she called me, she needed help and fast.

I started treating her to shift her lifestyle using therapeutics based on the ancient systems of Yoga and Ayurveda. After examining her and asking about her recent activities, I determined that she had poor digestion, which in turn led to toxic buildup on her skin. These digestive issues, along with constant work and travel, created too much heat in her body. I advised her to reduce the amount of food she was eating, take cooling herbs to curb the heat and other imbalances, and apply herbal remedies topically to reverse the dry itchy symptoms. Because of her commitment to her health, Maria adhered to this regimen. A week and a half later, she appeared at the Emmys free of rashes.

This story might seem like a nice advertisement for how an intense program can bring better health in very little time, but my purpose in sharing Maria's story has little to do with her work in preparing for the Emmys. When Maria realized how much more effective these methods were than all the medications she had used, she wanted to know everything she could about Ayurveda, Yoga, and the many ways this path could help her live a better life. Now that she enjoyed clear skin and had even lost a bit of weight, she wanted more.

Through our consultations, I found that Maria was inclined to suppress emotions that came up during her day. She pushed through to get things done instead of working out why she was reacting to whatever challenged her. This tendency, along with not breathing properly, was exacerbating the symptoms we had worked to resolve. To help her overcome these situations, we started integrating Yoga postures, breathing techniques, and other practices associated with the Yogic path. She began drinking hot water in the morning, eating only when hungry, and simplifying her life. Little by little, she went from using her asthma inhaler several times a day to not needing it at all. Her skin problems never came back. She lost ten pounds without even trying. In the first year that we worked together, not only did she improve her health, but her entire world began to shift. Her first book was a *New York Times* bestseller many times over, and she left her job as a correspondent at *Access Hollywood* to become a host of *Extra*. But more importantly, rather than allowing herself to repress the adverse emotions she felt throughout the day, Maria now had the tools to help her respond to those situations with a sense of groundedness and purpose. In one year's time, Maria was approaching her life in a completely different way.

The Potential

We've all encountered those books that promise a completely different life in no time. "Lose three dress sizes in thirty days!" "Find true happiness in two weeks!" But even though such programs are trendy today, it doesn't mean that they're helpful in the long term. These programs don't provide us with an effective way to stick with the changes we've implemented in that short amount of time. They promise us unrealistic results. Sure, we might succeed in getting a flatter tummy for a wedding or a trip to the beach, but what happens the following week? Do we maintain our health and happiness, or do we fall back into old patterns until there's another wedding to attend?

Most of us, of course, know the answer to these questions. We do fall back into those old patterns; health and happiness go away as quickly as our waistlines. To create real, lasting change throughout our lives, we must leave behind the thirty-day quick-fix solutions that let us down year after year and instead focus on one plan that will deliver lasting, life-changing results. We must embrace the possibility of a better life for ourselves. The One Plan is a full one-year program designed to provide a different approach to your life.

In 1501, a twenty-six-year-old Michelangelo petitioned members of the Florentine Office of Works for the opportunity to work on a sculpture. The job was to transform a nineteen-foot-tall block of marble known as "the Giant" into a sculpture commemorating the city's recent liberation from the book-burning rule of Girolamo Savonarola. Two sculptors had attempted to work on this immense marble over the course of the nearly hundred years since it was extracted. It had been poorly blocked with a huge gaping hole, and had been left exposed to the elements for decades. Despite the damage, Michelangelo saw the marble's potential. He used a steady hand to gradually strip the block of its nonessential pieces until—almost three years later—he revealed the Hebrew youth who had always been underneath. The result would be a source of joy to the world for many centuries to come, for the statue is what we now know as the *David*. This came to be because Michelangelo had a vision and allowed the statue to emerge in its own time.

What if you could uncover your greatest potential despite whatever damage you've endured over the years, and reveal your own masterpiece within? Wouldn't you want to find this reality for yourself?

And, most important, isn't your life worth more than thirty days?

The Problem

In the early part of my life, I worked as a fashion model. I participated in some of the most prominent campaigns of the 1980s and 1990s, including being the star of a three-season Guess Jeans campaign and the face of well-known labels like Versace. I even starred in Madonna's "Express Yourself" video. The life of a fashion model was just what you might imagine: I lived a life of travel, prestigious parties, shooting and filming in all the major cities of the world, enjoying late nights, and sleeping in until I fancied getting up. And while it might sound enjoyably luxurious, it wasn't allowing me to live a more purposeful life.

Early in this chapter of my life, I met a man named Ron. He had been a model back in the 1960s but had adopted a natural, simple life after being diagnosed with HIV. Under his guidance, I took my first Yoga workshops, read a stack of spiritual books, and began to consider that life could be more than runways and photo shoots.

Ron taught me the value of a life of purpose and spiritual growth. When he passed away in 2000, he didn't die in pain and sadness, like many who succumbed to AIDS; he had found contentment and peace. When he was no longer with me, I realized that he had been my mentor. I realized that a life of weight lifting, late-night indulgence, and constant luxury wasn't helping me find my purpose.

Since leaving my career in fashion, I've learned how to live healthier through the principles and methods of Ayurveda. I've learned that Yoga isn't simply an assortment of pretzel-like postures for gaining flexibility; it is an ancient, dynamic system of spiritual growth and personal development. I've devoted my life to practicing these ancient disciplines and helping others discover their full potential. Most of us lead almost entirely unnatural lives. We run on a treadmill instead of through fields. Instead of drinking water, we consume soft drinks sweetened with processed corn grown by giant corporations that genetically modify their crops. We use synthetic medications in an attempt to resolve our ailments, much like Maria did without success. We spend years in front of computer, TV, and smartphone screens.

But it doesn't have to be this way. In this book, I present a program that will help you use the ancient wisdom of Yoga and Ayurveda to create a healthier, more meaningful way of life. True change happens when we fit ourselves into a long-term plan, not when we fit a plan to our imbalanced, short-term desires.

The Plan

Many who are drawn to personal growth books collect an entire library: one book for exercise, one for diet, one for overcoming fear, one for creating better relationships, and one for spiritual growth. But the ancient sages of India observed that our bodies' relative health dictates the balance or imbalance of our minds. And the more imbalanced our minds, the farther we are from realizing genuine happiness in our lives. The One Plan won't provide piecemeal advice about components of your life; instead it will provide you with an ambitious but authentic lifestyle overhaul all in one program. It will help you resolve all sorts of issues that I've helped my clients with for years: physical complaints like obesity and fatigue, mental obstacles like anger and poor relationships, and spiritual challenges like a lack of purpose or fulfillment.

How is this possible? Ayurveda and Yoga, India's ancient systems of growth, are the oldest medical and spiritual systems in use today. They provide a blueprint for identifying the root cause of any imbalances we may experience. Maria may have been suffering from skin complaints, but she was also struggling to overcome obstacles in her professional life. She could have followed one program that promised her glowing skin in seven days and another that taught her to take charge of her work life, but instead she confronted the heated busyness of her life and everything fell into place all at once. The One Plan will help you identify the root cause of your physical, emotional, interpersonal, and professional challenges. Rather than merely treating a symptom, such as a skin outbreak or a problem at work, you will address your life as a whole. When all aspects of who you are become united, you experience the fulfillment and purpose you deserve.

The One Plan has been structured to shift you into a better life while allowing you time to do so through its yearlong format. Like Michelangelo chipping away at the Giant, you will change your lifestyle incrementally so that you aren't overwhelmed by the daunting task of removing harmful habits and choices from your life. You will clear out your cupboard of packaged foods one day, then clear out your bathroom the next. You'll breathe for five minutes one day, and five and a half the next. Bit by bit, you'll chip away at yourself until you are free of disease, less encumbered by strong emotions, and less likely to fall back into destructive patterns. Rather than pursuing a system that promises you light at the end of a tunnel, you will recognize that actually, the light is you.

In one year, your life will be different. With one program, you can make this change take place. You might have picked up this book to clear your skin of blemishes, to attract better relationships in your professional or personal life, or to find out why you were put on this earth in the first place. After you follow the One Plan, you will achieve all this and more.

You will have found your purpose.

one year to the real you

OUR JOURNEY ALONG THIS PATH BEGINS WITH TWO STORIES. THE first is about a man who suffered from chronic fatigue. In high school, he struggled to sustain his energy throughout the day. He experienced muscle fatigue, body aches, and sinus headaches. He woke up every morning feeling foggy-headed like he had a hangover. His doctor told him to get some rest and take some vitamin supplements. By the time he got to college, his condition had worsened.

Over the years, he went through many tests to determine why he always felt so run down. He was tested for allergies, blood disorders, and vitamin and mineral deficiencies—but all the tests came back negative. He hoped to improve his sleep by having surgery on a deviated septum. That didn't help either. At one point, a doctor diagnosed him as having clinical depression and prescribed Adderall; after a month on that, he felt jittery and awful. By the time he came to me—about fifteen years after he first struggled with this problem—he had lost faith in Western doctors.

During our first consultation, I examined him and determined that there were imbalances throughout his body, including some hardness in the small intestine. I prescribed herbs to help get his energy up and had him give his entire diet an overhaul. He subsisted primarily on processed foods, including cold cereal, pasta, chocolate, and frozen vegetables. I had him change his diet to whole, fresh foods, eating until his stomach felt half full. He wasn't allowed leftovers or microwaved foods. Previously, he drank four cups of coffee a day to keep his energy up. I had him quit coffee the first day.

The first few days of his overhaul went exactly as you might imagine. He struggled to eat whole foods every day and had a hard time eating smaller meals. Caffeine withdrawal made him feel sicker than he had in a long time. But by the fifth day, he felt better. After a week, his energy started to increase. He wasn't as foggy in the morning. Each day, he felt a little clearer in the head, his muscles ached a little less, and his headaches were less severe. He had previously needed to take a nap most afternoons just to make it through the day, and now naps were no longer necessary. Eventually, he started to wake up with plenty of energy and sustain that energy throughout the day.

This transformation took place in three weeks.

The second story involves a man who felt stuck in his life. After a short career as a public school chemistry teacher, he realized that his greatest passion was film. He decided to set out for Los Angeles to become a film director. Thanks to his connections, he was able to land several jobs as a production assistant. He took some acting workshops to learn how to better connect with actors on set. Eventually, he worked his way up to assistant directing—but that's where his upward mobility stopped.

Though he was getting by, he wasn't achieving his ultimate goal of directing films. He believed that the best first step toward becoming a director was to write a screenplay that he could produce. But he wasn't writing any screenplays. Not even close.

I visited my new client in his home to help him get his life back on track. When I arrived, I took a look around the living room and saw a desk and a chair, a couch, and other living room furniture . . . and stuff everywhere.

He had Post-its reminding him of all sorts of things—ideas for new projects as well as tasks for his everyday life. He had outlines posted to the walls in case he wanted to write down thoughts on the spot. He had piles of library books that he kept renewing over and over in the hope that he would eventually read them. He had tools for filmmaking stacked up in a closet. He was a practicing Buddhist and chanted several times a week—but even his chanting space was cluttered with a dry-erase board and more stuff.

I took a look at this space—the piles, the clutter, and the disarray—and told him that I had no idea what the person who lived there did for a living. It certainly didn't make me think that it was a person who took screenwriting seriously.

My new client felt stuck in his career as a filmmaker because he wasn't writing. But with so much stuff everywhere, it was no surprise that he was distracted. I had him clear out his house, getting rid of the Post-its, outlines, library books, film supplies, and anything else that wasn't immediately necessary for daily life. If he cleared it all out, then perhaps he would have greater clarity when he sat down to write and would start getting some screenplays completed. I had him increase his commitment to his chanting practice, for though he did chant, he did so only for a couple of minutes sporadically throughout the week. More discipline in his practice would give him greater discipline in all his endeavors—including screenwriting.

Unfortunately, even with all of the clutter gone and a regular chanting practice, he still couldn't focus on his writing. After several weeks of working with him, I decided we needed to reassess. "You still haven't made any progress with your writing," I said.

"Nope," he said. I considered this for a moment. He said this matter-of-factly, without any real disappointment.

"But do you even like writing?" I finally said.

"Of course I don't like writing," he said. "Getting something down on paper is like pulling teeth."

"So why are you doing it?"

"Well, it's sort of a means to an end. If I want to direct, then I've got to write something that can be directed."

I considered this, but then remembered that writing and directing weren't the only ways he had approached his new career.

"And what about your acting workshops?" I asked him.

"What about them?"

"Did you enjoy that work?"

"Well, sure," he said, "but it wasn't really like work per se."

"Why not?"

My client then told me that he often received positive feedback from his acting teachers, fellow classmates, and people he worked with during various acting jobs. They all talked about his natural presence as an actor.

"I never even thought of acting as work," he said. "It was something that just seemed to make sense to me."

"Mmm," I said.

He looked at me, waiting for me to say more. When I didn't, he looked around at his recently tidied space.

"I shouldn't be writing, should I?"

"Is writing the only way to be part of a film?" I asked.

"No, I guess it isn't," he said.

I then suggested that he not only keep his home free of clutter, but that he free himself of writing—the career track that he didn't need.

After that conversation, he signed up for a class on the business of acting. A friend of his cut a reel of footage he had done the previous year, and he assembled a list of agents and managers to whom he could submit the reel and a list of ten TV shows that featured the types of characters that he would be good for. He had previously thought that acting wasn't a viable career, but now he was doing whatever he could to make this career a reality. Writing a screenplay may have been like pulling teeth, but taking actionable steps toward an acting career came as naturally as acting itself.

You may have noticed that these stories are very different: one is about a man who experienced physical problems like chronic fatigue and headaches, and the other involves a man who felt stuck in his career. One story is about struggling in the body, and the other is about struggling in the mind.

And yet, these two stories are about the same man.

Body and Mind: Inexorably Linked

The two stories focus on Christian, who was cast on my TV show *A Model Guru*. The work we did together was part of the show, in which I worked with people who were struggling with debilitating illness, helping them make over their lives through practices found in Yoga and Ayurveda.

I told Christian's story as two separate narratives to make a point: whether our struggles are related to our bodies or our minds, whatever happens with one inevitably affects the other. Christian had a particularly hard time with chronic fatigue: he could barely sustain his energy level through the day. He was also holding his career prisoner by remaining stuck in a mind-set about what he needed to do. Was his fatigue undermining his clarity about his career? Of course. Was his lack of clarity exacerbating his fatigue? Most definitely.

The principles and methods outlined in this book teach us to address the root cause of the struggles or setbacks we face in life. If our bodies are diseased, we have to also look at mental issues that might be holding us back. If we feel stuck in a mindset or are struggling to figure out some aspect of our lives, we have to also address diet, sleep, and other physical considerations. Modern medicine teaches us to compartmentalize our health. As a result, it is common to consider diet as one contained aspect of our lives and mental health as another aspect, never imagining that something as basic as the clutter in our houses could cause the setbacks we've encountered. But when Christian no longer allowed himself to be bogged down by his illness, he was able to rid himself of an unnecessary approach to his career. His story teaches us that doing something as simple as clearing up clutter and returning library books can instigate a clarity that opens up our lives to new and exciting possibilities.

Since you have picked up this book, you are probably open to the possibility that you can improve your life. You might not know what that life will look like, but you at least think that something better is possible. You might have an illness that has plagued you for many years, like Christian did, and you would like to improve how you feel. Perhaps you feel that this book will help you lose weight, or that you'll attract better relationships, or that you'll figure out what you want to do with your life. Perhaps when you first picked up this book, you allowed yourself to hope for a moment that there really is something more to life than filling it with one distraction after another. Perhaps you thought that the program in this book would give you the answers you're looking for.

And you would be right.

This change won't come easy, though. Those of us who live in the modern world are inundated with obligations and distractions on any given day, and it would be *so much easier* if we could make our bodies and minds feel better by taking a magic pill and then continuing on with our lives as usual. We would no longer have that pain in our lower back. We would no longer feel stressed all the time. We would feel good.

But as you already know, this program is not about taking a magic pill. It's about making a substantial shift in your life over time. Since you're willing to consider this admittedly lengthy journey, you must also believe you are worth the time and effort necessary for creating such a shift in your life. And you certainly are. But rather than settling for getting rid of lower back pain or feeling a bit less stressed, the One Plan will show you how to enrich your entire state of being. You will see that there truly is a beauty within you waiting to be revealed.

But before we unveil this masterpiece to the world, we must address a basic issue we all face. We must understand the reason why our bodies, minds, and everything else about our situations are not in the condition we want them to be in.

Our Struggle

When you were a child, did you ever want something for yourself—an ice cream cone, a puppy, or even greater respect from an older sibling—but weren't able to get it? Did your parents tell you no, or did your diminutive size make commanding respect an almost impossible task? What did you say to yourself in response to those situations? Did you say, "Oh, well, I'm happy to not have any ice cream at all" and then carry on with your day with a smile on your face? If you did, you'd probably be the first child ever to have done so. More likely, you got upset and threw a fit. You may have thought something like this: "When I'm older, things will be different. That's when I'll get whatever I want."

You didn't like the situation you were in, and you believed that being older (and, of course, bigger) would get you that ice cream cone, a puppy, and everything else your heart desired. But did that reality ever come true? As an adult, maybe you can get an ice cream cone if you feel like it, but are you satisfied with all aspects of your life, like that child who expected to have whatever he or she wanted? Is every workday filled with perfect moments, or do you experience stress about deadlines or tension related to coworkers? Are you in a perfect relationship that makes you happy all the time, or are there times when you struggle to communicate effectively—if you're even in a relationship at all? Has every aspect of your life fallen into place now that you're old enough to get a puppy if you want one?

Though things may be different now that you're older, my guess is that they've not all fallen into place for you. In fact, every person in the history of the planet—myself included—has struggled to get things to fall into place in a way that makes every moment enjoyable or even bearable. And this struggle that each of us experiences happens for one very simple reason: we struggle in life because we suffer.

Suffering is a word that is likely familiar to you. You've no doubt used it many times before, perhaps when describing how you felt when you were sick with the flu for five days, or when you think of the many millions of people around the world who live in extreme poverty. But it also accounts for why we experience chronic fatigue, stress, fear, or general unhappiness. We experience all these things because we suffer in body and mind.

In the traditions that underpin the One Plan, the simplest way to define the word *suffering* is to equate it with pain. We have pain in the body, and we have pain in the mind. Given this definition, you can probably envision how we suffer physically in the body. We accept physical pain and discomfort as part of life: soreness, inflammation, stiffness, tiredness, and achiness. We experience physical pain when we're sick, when we're burdened with disease, and when something in our bodies is damaged (like a broken bone). In looking at Christian's story, it's easy enough to see how he suffered physically. He felt foggy, tired, and fatigued for much of the day. Maria experienced rashes. When we suffer physically, we experience an imbalance that keeps us from feeling healthy, fit, and ready to take on whatever comes our way.

But what do you imagine when you think of pain in the mind? Perhaps you think of day-to-day stress, or grief after the loss of a loved one. Though stress does relate to pain in the mind, as do strong emotions like grief, mental suffering includes a much larger issue: We suffer in the mind whenever we rely on the world beyond ourselves to make us happy—or when we blame it for our unhappiness.

This is what happened when we were young and didn't get what we wanted. We promised ourselves that things would be different when we were older and bigger. Though most of us have graduated from ice cream cones and puppies, we still hold the outside world accountable for our happiness. When we say to ourselves that we will be happy when we finally make a lot of money, we are holding money responsible for the fulfillment we currently lack. When we tell ourselves that we are miserable because our spouses don't understand us or don't do nice things for us, we are holding them responsible for our lives not being the ideal they should be. Every day, we crave more stuff, more pleasure, more excitement, more relationships, and more comfortable circumstances. Every day, we take offense at rudeness directed toward us, come down on ourselves for mistakes we make, hold on to conflicts from the past, and brace ourselves for setbacks in the future.

You might be thinking, "So what if I do wish I had more money or blame my misery on an insensitive spouse? Isn't that just the way life goes?" When we have this type of relationship to the outside world, we are vulnerable to its fickleness. Yes, we might feel happy when we suddenly get a windfall of cash, but does that happiness last forever? What if the money were stolen from us, and we suddenly had nothing again? The money that so recently brought us joy now brings us immense pain. We think that having a relationship will solve all our problems, but relationships often seem to cause more problems than they solve. When we rely on an object, situation, incident, or opportunity to make us happy, we open ourselves up to disappointment when it doesn't happen. Then, as a result of this disappointment, we react with painful emotions, like anger ("How dare you say that to me!"), sadness ("Now my money is all gone"), grief ("I've never felt so alone"), worry ("Why hasn't he called yet?"), and perhaps most significantly, fear ("What if my life never becomes what I want it to be?"). When we feel such painful emotions, we experience turmoil. It is here, in this state of pain, that we suffer in the mind.

Anyone who has taken a psychology course or read about a classic rock band's tragic breakup is familiar with the term *ego*. When we react adversely to situations that don't go the way we want them to—when we experience pain in the mind—we are allowing our ego to control us. The ego is an aspect of the mind that acts like a tyrannical little dictator who needs total control of everything. Just like a dictator sets out to take over other countries and build an empire that gives power over the masses, our ego needs to control everything that surrounds us on behalf of an ever-increasing need for gratification. It's what makes us want to be better than other people at sports, to have the biggest house on the street, to win other people's attention and praise, and to generally think that we're better than others. Though no dictator has ever conquered the entire planet, what would happen if one did? If the only thing that validates a dictator's power is ever-increasing control over his surroundings, what would he do when placing that last flag on that last piece of land? Would he take to space travel and conquer uninhabited planets? The idea of that is absurd, and spending our lives trying to gratify our ego is also absurd. Our ego wants to control everything around us, but with billions of people, trillions upon trillions of plants and animals, ever-changing weather, and the unpredictability of any given moment of any given day, it's unlikely that the entire world will ever be controlled by anyone. With trillions of ways for us to be influenced and affected by the world, there are just as many opportunities for us to react out of anger, fear, or other difficult emotions. This makes the ego not only useless but the cause of our mental pain.

Christian may have suffered a great deal from his chronic fatigue, but he also suffered mentally from his failure to achieve success as a filmmaker. In letting go of his need to write screenplays, he let go of his ego's need for validation through what he thought was the only appropriate way to participate in the film industry. When he abandoned the need for that validation, he no longer experienced disappointment in not receiving it. And without that disappointment, he was open to pursue other endeavors that were more intrinsically satisfying to him. By adjusting his mind-set to favor his natural talents, Christian began to confront his suffering in the mind.

Given that body and mind are inexorably linked, what affects one inevitably affects the other. Suffering in the body ("I feel achy all over, and it's hard to get out of bed") leads to suffering in the mind ("I'm not doing enough with my life"). Eventually, life fills with pain rather than serving as a source of happiness and fulfillment.

Living in Love

In 2011, I was asked to participate in the Newark Peace Education Summit. This conference took place in Newark, New Jersey, over the course of a weekend and was founded and resided over by His Holiness the Dalai Lama as well as numerous other leaders and activists. The purpose of the summit was to create greater awareness of peace-building efforts and teach attendees about projects in support of nonviolent practices. The heart of this event was a series of panel discussions held in the conference center's auditorium.

As well as teaching Yoga and meditation at the summit, I also attended several panel discussions. The first included people from different backgrounds, including Nobel Peace Prize laureates Jody Williams and Shirin Ebadi, author Deepak Chopra, and renowned spiritual scholar Robert Thurman. Rabbi Michael Lerner led the room in a song of peace. About twenty minutes into the panel, His Holiness the Dalai Lama came onstage accompanied by his translator. Through the beginning of the panel, the audience had maintained its interest and seemed to appreciate the ideas and philosophies being shared. But when His Holiness came onstage, everyone jumped to their feet and burst into applause. The entire room was filled with warmth and happiness. This sudden movement in energy felt sort of like an amphitheater when a rock star comes onstage after the audience has enjoyed the concert's opening act. But I didn't tell this story to describe this rock star reception. What struck me about His Holiness's entrance was not the enthusiasm of the applause but what happened after everyone settled down and returned to their seats: the warmth and happiness remained.

A boy named Lhamo Dondrub—eventually renamed Tenzin Gyatso—was selected as the fourteenth Dalai Lama when he was only two years old. He was formally recognized as such when he was fifteen. Because of this early responsibility, he has spent his entire life advocating for the rights of his native country of Tibet and teaching Tibetan Buddhism to the world. His devotion to this path has empowered him to be a messenger of peace and compassion, but it also has shaped the presence he emanates. That day at the Newark Peace Education Summit, His Holiness the Dalai Lama walked onstage and elevated an entire room to a higher state.

Each of us is born a natural being, just like flowers, birds, and every other living thing in existence. As part of this natural order of life, we each have the potential to embody this perfection throughout our time on earth. While the perfection of flowers and hummingbirds shows in the way they bloom or fly, our perfection manifests as our capacity for joy. When we chip away at the discomfort in our bodies and our enslavement to the ego in our minds, we create a state of supreme balance. We exist as perfect, natural beings. This entity within each of us—this element of nature—is known as the spirit.

The goal of spiritual growth is to end the suffering in our bodies and minds so that we may be guided by the spirit and reveal its natural perfection. When we end our suffering, we manifest the divine light that exists in all living things. We may call this presence nature, God, or, as it will be referred to in this book, the Creative Spirit or just the Spirit. In this spiritually realized state, we don't feel pain anywhere in our bodies. We don't suffer from any turmoil or other affliction of the ego. When we are alone, considering the struggles that have happened or the uncertainty of what is to come, we feel neither bitter about the past nor frightened of the future. Instead, we experience the world as we are meant to experience it, enjoying the richest possibilities for our lives and our greatest potential.

When the Dalai Lama entered that auditorium in Newark, he gave this perfection to everyone out of a love for all humanity. And the people in that room offered their love in return.

A Spiritual Practice

Imagine what would happen if someone gave you a set of golf clubs as a gift. It's a very professional-looking set, and since you've never golfed before you enjoy taking out the various drivers, irons, and other clubs and inspecting them. You even buy a book to introduce you to the sport and read it cover to cover. But the set of clubs finds its way into your garage, and you never take it to a golf course. In receiving these clubs as a gift and reading a book, you may have become more aware of the sport, but have you actually participated in it? Of course the answer to this question is no—talking about golf, reading about golf, and even owning a set of clubs in no way means you're playing the game. Not even a bit.

The same can be said of spiritual growth. We might like the prospect of resolving physical and mental suffering or the idea of filling an auditorium with love, but how many of us actually set out to create a life in which those things will happen? How many of us own golf clubs, so to speak, without actually going to a course and swinging them around?

A system of spiritual growth, be it the Tibetan Buddhist discipline taught by the Dalai Lama or the one outlined in this book, may be followed by anyone seeking greater health and joy in life. Each path requires us to commit to specific behaviors and routines that will aid us as we attempt to liberate our minds from the ego and live in contentment and peace. If we were to pursue this lifestyle with devotion for many years, we would attain a state in which we have fully awakened our spirit and emanate its perfection in every aspect of our lives. This state of being is known by various terms—enlightenment, salvation, nirvana, or something else. Since this state reflects full realization of our individual spirit, in this book we will refer to it as *self-realization*.

In Christian's story, he had to go through lifestyle modifications, routines, and rituals to increase his energy and shift his mind-set. But when I spoke to him, he was not particularly interested in fully realizing his spirit. As a practicing Buddhist, he was aware of that possibility, but he mostly just wanted to commit himself to a lifestyle that gave him more energy and greater focus. Even the Dalai Lama, who offers so much love, has said he is unsure of his own grasp of the methods he is using. But regardless of whether we want to heal our bodies and improve our minds or truly invest in a life that takes us to a heightened state of being, we ultimately need to not just own the clubs but learn to use them too.

The only way for us to shift our lifestyle and find our way out of suffering is to set an intention to change and then follow with daily actions to make that change a reality. These actions are collectively known as a *spiritual practice,* or simply a *practice.* Buying a book like this and reading it is a great first step. But if you don't put the book down and practice the methods it has taught you, then you haven't done anything more than become aware of pain in your body and mind.

Patanjali and the Eightfold Path

The One Plan is based on the ancient systems of Yoga and Ayurveda. It follows a tradition that was laid out for us over two thousand years ago by an Indian sage named Patanjali. It is a system called the Eightfold Path.

A number of spiritual texts have greatly influenced the Indian spiritual tradition, including the Vedas, a series of texts that are said to have been directly manifested from a divine source, and the Upanishads, an ancient text that forms the basis of many Hindu traditions. But Patanjali authored a particularly influential text that forms the basis of the One Plan: the Yoga Sutras.

This text forms the basis of everything we associate with Yoga today: postures, breathing practices, meditation practices, chanting, and other practices that relate to how we behave in our day-to-day lives. Every Yoga studio you've walked past, every ashram you've read about, and every Yoga DVD you see in the store are all in some way based on the nonreligious work that Patanjali produced over two thousand years ago.

Though we don't know much about Patanjali, he is thought by many scholars to have lived a little over two thousand years ago and is regarded as the possible author of other significant texts as well. And though he was a physical being who lived on earth for a set period of time, he is regarded as a pure manifestation of divine light who came into being to serve humanity. This gave him an intuitive grasp of the message of the Creative Spirit, and it is through this divine authority that Patanjali authored the Yoga Sutras.

Composed of 196 aphorisms, the Sutras are an incredibly brief text. And yet, all of the Yoga practices done through ashrams, studios, and DVDs can be summed up by the second aphorism:

"Chitta vritti nirodhah."

This bit of Sanskrit defines Yoga as a system for relieving the suffering of the mind. When we relieve this suffering, we no longer react to the moment with painful emotions but rather observe our thoughts and allow the world to unfold exactly as it needs to without our ego initiating the need for control. We empower ourselves to encounter seemingly adverse situations and, rather than feel pain, we may use the experience as an opportunity for growth. This sentence tells us that the entirety of the Yogic tradition is about training the mind to let go of the story our ego tells in response to a situation that causes painful emotions like anger and fear.

There are, of course, many paths of Yoga. There's Bhakti Yoga, the path of devotion. There's Karma Yoga, the path of selfless service. There's Jnana Yoga, the path of self-study. The list goes on, and there are various disciplines within each of these paths. What is important, though, is that every one of these paths serves the same purpose. Each path requires the participant to commit to a spiritual practice.

In the Yoga Sutras, Patanjali explains the Eightfold Path, an eight-step system for working toward self-realization. This system is also known as *Raja* or the Royal Path, a reference to the mind's dominance over our state of being. When we master our minds, we attain the highest or royal quality of life.

Patanjali teaches that we must pursue all components of the Eightfold Path, and in order. After taking one step, we move on to the next one. Through this sequential format, the Sutras provide readers with a compass for navigating what can often seem like a daunting task. Eventually, we will no longer be swayed by our ego's need for control. We will no longer need to make more money to be happy, or require people to act in a particular way to end our lack of happiness. We will rely on our inner peace to create a life of fulfillment and purpose.

Typically, when someone in Western culture decides to start practicing Yoga, they seek out someplace to practice the physical postures that most people in the modern world associate with this tradition. According to Patanjali, though, not only are postures not the entirety of this tradition, but they're not even the first step.

The first two steps of Patanjali's eight-step system address our day-to-day behaviors, much like the Ten Commandments in Judeo-Christianity and the Noble Eightfold Path in Buddhism. They are:

- THE ABSTENTIONS (*yamas*): five acts of avoiding behaviors that perpetuate our personal suffering.

- THE OBSERVATIONS (*niyamas*): five balancing behaviors pursued for greater peace.

The middle steps take us through practices that are more typically associated with Yogic tradition, like postures and breathing. They include:

- POSTURES (*asana*): stretching and strengthening the body to be able to sit with greater ease for hours at a time.

- BREATH CONTROL (*pranayama*): using the breath to shift the mind out of an emotional state.

- SENSE CONTROL (*pratyahara*): shifting how the senses react to objects in the outside world so that they no longer encumber the mind.

- CONCENTRATION (*dharana*): focusing the mind on a single object so as to train it to no longer respond to the ego's stories.

And the final steps of the path take us into the state of self-realization:

- MEDITATION (*dhyana*): getting the mind to let go of thoughts, free itself of emotional burdens, and attain a state of equanimity.

- SAMADHI: complete and total absorption in the spirit—an existence of total bliss.

When approached as a whole system, the Eightfold Path provides an opportunity to resolve pain and discomfort in our bodies, then resolve imbalances in our minds, and finally, should we choose to pursue it at a more heightened level, to ultimately realize and reveal our spirit. Here, in this program, I provide the tools to create that experience for yourself.

getting started with the one plan

THE ONE PLAN FOLLOWS A FIFTY-TWO-WEEK STRUCTURE. IT WILL show you what to do every day of those fifty-two weeks, and through this pursuit you will be empowered to discover how best to live. The book is intended to provide a blueprint for gradually working your way to a healthier, more beneficial life without overwhelming your schedule or overly compromising aspects of your life that are at odds with those high-minded ideals. Just like Michelangelo would never have taken the sixteenth-century equivalent of a sledgehammer to a piece of marble to get his process started, neither will you be expected to sit for hours on the first day to find a state of self-realization.

Patanjali calls on us to pursue the eight steps of this path in sequence, and that's exactly what the fifty-two-week structure of the One Plan does. First you will pursue the abstentions and observations of the first two steps, and then you will move on to postures, breath control, and so on. I've organized this program to be true to Patanjali's message while also being attainable within your modern, fast-paced life. But how does this happen?

To return to the golf analogy, if you were to take those clubs out to a driving range and knock a few balls around, would you expect to be hitting them straight and long right from the start? If you went to an actual golf course, would you expect to play like Tiger Woods? Just like you would have to actually use the clubs to learn how to play, you would have to first develop the fundamentals of a golf swing before you work on distance and power. You would have to eliminate your need for a handicap before you joined the PGA Tour.

Using Yoga and Ayurveda to create a life of greater love and happiness is like starting off with the fundamentals of a golf swing and working our way up to playing with the pros in the US Open. We have already explored the terms *body, mind,* and *spirit,* and these three entities play a crucial role in helping us determine how to best pursue the high ideals of the Yogic path as a whole.

The Three Realms

For each of the fifty-two weeks that compose this program, I provide specific exercises to help you craft a daily routine. Each component has been divided into three realms: the realm of the body, the realm of the mind, and the realm of the spirit. When you start any given week of the program, you will be given the choice of which realm to pursue. This choice will depend on whether you are just getting started on your journey or whether you've been working on this for years.

The *realm of the body* is the first step of any given practice. This realm is defined by the physical aspects of our existence, like the health and condition of the body and the way we interact with the physical space around us. Just like Michelangelo took a mallet and chisel to the block of marble to knock off larger chunks to give the sculpture its basic shape, we first pursue physical aspects of the practice as the largest, broadest strokes before delving into the more subtle workings of the mind. One of the abstentions we will explore is nonviolence, the act of avoiding behaviors that do harm to ourselves and others. We start this work in the realm of the body, which means that we abstain from physical forms of violence like yelling and consuming harmful foods and substances. Once we've worked through the realm of the body, our bodies become healthy and our relationship to the physical world becomes more balanced.

The *realm of the mind* is the second step of any given practice. This realm is defined by the mental aspects of our existence, like the extent to which our thoughts are dictated by the ego's need for control, and whether our emotions are troubled or more fulfilling. Once Michelangelo had finished the rougher step of knocking off large pieces of marble, he then began using tools similar to today's rasps and rifflers to refine the sculpture and give it its final form. Similarly, finding a state of physical balance empowers us to achieve greater balance in the mind. After we have successfully practiced the physical aspects of nonviolence, we work on avoiding harmful thoughts about ourselves and others. This allows us to respond to adversity with greater calm and peace. When we attain balance in the mind, we no longer suffer from life's unexpected developments.

The *realm of the spirit,* the highest realm, embodies the perfection to which this path aspires. This is the realm in which a person exhibits love for all living things and sees others as themselves—for all are connected through the same divine source. For most of us, the concepts and practices related to the realm of the spirit may seem daunting and even esoteric. But that's really okay. Once we have succeeded in working through the realms of the body and the mind, working toward that state of being is simply the natural next step. When a person pursues the spiritual realm of their nonviolence practice, they love all people—even those who exhibit violence toward them and others. To create this love is to shine one's light onto others. Thus Michelangelo used the finest tools to polish the marble so that its shiny surface would glow.

As you pursue any given aspect of this program, be it the two weeks devoted to nonviolence or the eight weeks devoted to postures, you will be given a series of tasks to pursue in the realm that will most benefit you, given where you are in your life at that moment. You may find that you are best suited to practice entirely within one realm, as will certainly be the case if you are just starting out, or you may decide to pick and choose among several. Because of the ego's desire for control, you may be tempted to compete with yourself and qualify the value of your experience by how quickly you work your way through everything. But if you are to truly benefit from the concepts and practices laid out in this program, you must master one realm before you move on to the next so as to receive the greatest possible benefit.

Good Morning, Sunshine

When you wake up in the morning, how do you typically feel? Do you look forward to a brand-new day and start singing along with the birds in the trees, or do you press the snooze button for thirty minutes, stagger out of bed, and rush through a morning ritual involving a hurried shower and two (or three) cups of coffee? For those of us who struggle with our health and well-being, getting going in the morning can be the most difficult task of the day. But allowing mornings to be bogged down with lethargy and addictive stimulants sets a tone for the rest of the day: rather than an opportunity to find our purpose, each day is something to survive.

The One Plan is designed to help you create a better life for yourself, first by establishing a more productive and satisfying tone for your morning. In the program, you will craft a morning routine of reflection and rituals that will nourish your body and mind. When you give yourself just a few minutes each morning to take care of yourself, you will start to see the value of your time during the rest of the day and feel more content with each moment. Soon your days will no longer be something to be merely survived, but rather a time to be relished.

The Presence Practice

A key component of your new morning routine will be an exercise I call the Presence Practice. Many disciplines in this program are simple enough to pursue incrementally—whether it's extending the amount of time between eating and going to bed or gradually adding minutes to a breathing practice. However, some practices found in the One Plan, especially in the first twenty weeks, are more challenging to measure. Abstaining from violence or dishonesty might be part of the groundwork for building a solid foundation, but how does one pursue these goals incrementally? Tell the truth three times one day, and then four times the next? Use four curse words at the guy who cut you off on the highway one day, then only use three curse words a week later? Of course not. That would be less like spiritual growth and more like a really bad reality TV show.

Each of us has different obstacles to overcome and different behaviors we'd like to change, so it would be presumptuous of me to think that all people will benefit from doing *exactly* the same thing. Though the basis of this program is formulaic, following it by no means depends on everyone completing the same specific tasks in all aspects of their lives. Instead, I provide a basic template for you to use in applying many of the practices included in this program.

Anytime we are presented with the task of shifting a behavior, be it refraining from biting our nails or quitting smoking, we must do three things:

1. Recognize that there's an issue to be resolved ("I bite my nails even though I shouldn't").

2. Decide that we will work on the issue ("I will no longer bite my nails").

3. Act on the issue ("I'm nervous and am going to bite my nails— oh wait, I'm not doing that anymore").

The dentist once told me that I was causing mouth sores and gum problems for myself because I was chewing on the inside of my cheek. Though it was an effort, I learned to keep myself from continuing in that habit because I recognized that I had started it by mimicking my mother, decided to change it, and acted on that decision. This is what I call the Presence Practice. It is a process that requires us to be present to a certain behavior for a set period of time and to continually remind ourselves to shift that behavior. To change my cheek-chewing habit, I made this habit the absolute top priority in my day-to-day life for a set amount of time until the habit was gone.

The Presence Practice will be a key tool as you change your behaviors through the One Plan. For example, let's say that you are practicing truthfulness in Weeks 3–4 of the program. You may have discovered that you have someone in your life that you consider a friend but never want to spend time with. When she invites you to go somewhere, you tell her that you're super busy or that you're not feeling so hot. At no point, though, have you told her the truth: that you're not that busy and that you feel fine. You avoid spending time with her because you don't enjoy her company. You don't tell her how you really feel, though, because it's hard to hurt someone's feelings like that.

If you really don't enjoy the time you spend with this friend, then the pursuit of truthfulness will compel you to be honest with her: "I'd prefer to spend some time apart for right now, because I feel I'm in a different space than I once was." Or you may decide that you prefer for her to remain in your life, so you accept her invitations and enjoy her company for what it is.

Making a decision like this doesn't require two weeks of incremental work, as building up to a fifteen-minute breathing practice does. But though this sort of work isn't time-consuming, it certainly requires an investment of energy, thought, and emotions. And once you make this one decision, you will notice other areas of your life in which you are not being truthful.

How will you structure your pursuit of these behavioral changes? Throughout the first twenty weeks of the program—and even several times in the remaining thirty-two weeks—you will be asked to use the Presence Practice to change certain behaviors. This could be a behavior that's subtle or even internal, such as spending time with someone whose company you don't enjoy, or it could be something simple and overt, such as not repressing burps or stifling yawns. For subtle behaviors, we might have to go through a process of self-inquiry ("Do I have friends in my life with whom I'm not particularly fond of spending time?"), but for the simpler behaviors there's no self-inquiry involved ("Oh, I definitely suppress yawns when I talk to people so they don't think I'm rude; I will stop doing that"). For the subtle behaviors, I present a list of questions you may ask yourself as part of the practice—such as the one about having friends you aren't fond of spending time with. For simple behaviors, I'll just give you changes to make and you'll use the Presence Practice in the morning to alter that behavior.

Each morning after you wake up but before you start work, school, or whatever else you will be doing to fill your day, you are to find a quiet corner of your home, sit for five minutes in silence, and remind yourself to shift a behavior. When you need to engage in a process of self-inquiry, your task is to follow these steps:

1. Take the list of questions with you to your chosen sitting place. For the time you're sitting, you can either use a chair or sit on a cushion on the floor, but be sure to keep an upright spine. You may keep your eyes open or closed, but closing them will help shut out any activity going on around you.

2. Choose a question from the list that you think might be relevant, and ask yourself this question.

3. See what thoughts, memories, or perspectives come up in response to this question over the course of five minutes.

4. When you identify yourself as exhibiting a behavior ("I don't like spending time with that friend"), your task is to address that behavior by the end of the week.

5. If, by the end of the week, you haven't encountered a situation in which to address that behavior ("I will let her know that I'd prefer to spend some time apart right now"), create that opportunity before moving on to the next week ("I will give her a call").

6. If you finish reversing one behavior before the end of the week, go on to another question from the list.

7. Repeat this process in any subsequent weeks devoted to the same practice. (Since a Presence Practice on truthfulness is featured in Weeks 3 and 4, you will reverse at least one behavior for Week 3, and at least one behavior for Week 4.)

For each simple behavior you are to reverse, such as stifling yawns, simply sit for five minutes while reminding yourself to no longer behave in that way. Throughout the week, you are to remind yourself whenever the behavior comes up. When the week is up, continue maintaining an honest separation from the former friend, allowing yourself to yawn, or whatever else you have worked on.

The Presence Practice will help remind you that these behavioral shifts are valuable in the bigger picture of your life. Some days, you might have no success in being truthful about something, but other days it might seem like everything on this new path is aligning perfectly for you. But no matter what happens, by spending just five minutes a day focusing on the behaviors you seek to change and then creating the change in a tangible way by the end of the week, you'll be spending more time than you probably ever have on improving. And this is a start.

Building Bit by Bit for a Year

The format of the One Plan will allow you to take on a manageable amount of change at one time so that by the end of your year of work you will be in a completely different space. You will spend the first two weeks practicing non-violence, then add those practices to a practice of truthfulness (Weeks 3–4), continuing to build one practice on top of the previous one. Each section features an explanation of the concepts at hand, an overview of how the concepts relate to the three realms, the exercises and behaviors you will begin to incorporate into your lifestyle, and a recap providing you with an overview of your routine for those weeks.

As you work your way through the One Plan, always remember that though its concepts have been expressed in a way that keeps the modern-day practitioner in mind, it is still ultimately a two-thousand-year-old tradition that has proven valuable and beneficial for generations of seekers. The ancient sages of India set out a vision for how we may infuse our lives with balance, peace, and purpose. Patanjali consolidated this vision into a program we could all understand.

Now all you have to do is begin.

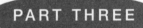

grounding
your
practice

HAVE YOU EVER SEEN CONSTRUCTION WORKERS LABORING OVER the early stages of building a house? After the land has been leveled and the bulldozers have cleared off, you might see them laying cinder blocks, pouring concrete, or making some other effort for weeks on end. Then, all of a sudden, walls sprout up out of nowhere. One day the house just looks like a submerged bit of concrete, and the next day it looks like . . . a house. There are beams. There are headers. There are door frames and window frames. Though there is still a lot to be done, you wonder why it took so long to get to this point given how fast this latest step is going.

This happens because laying a foundation, though it may not look like much work, it is actually an involved process that must be done with precision. If the foundation isn't level, the house will be lopsided. If the beams aren't poured correctly, the basement will be susceptible to flooding. Without careful preparation of the house's foundation, the house might as well not even be built for all the structural issues it will have.

The same is true of building a lifestyle around Yogic principles and ridding ourselves of suffering in the body and mind. We're far less likely to remain committed to a routine if we don't first have a personal investment in reforming our lifestyle. In the first two steps of the Eightfold Path, Patanjali has provided an opportunity to ground ourselves in productive intentions by altering our behavior throughout the day. These first two steps help shape our relationship to the world around us. Just as Maria didn't realize how much tension she held in her body in reaction to stressful situations, we often exhibit unproductive behaviors out of habit. These reactions can affect our health and happiness in a significant way and need to be controlled before we move on to the higher practices.

Patanjali starts us off not with physical postures or breathing, but with what he calls the abstentions (*yamas*) and the observations (*niyamas*). Postures, breathing, and the higher practices of this path are techniques that we pursue for a specific amount of time each day—like an exercise regimen. The abstentions and observations are behavioral guidelines that we follow all day long, and that eventually influence how we think and act. Patanjali presents ten practices (five abstentions and five observations) to incorporate into our lifestyle as we work to end our personal suffering. When we are successful, the foundation we lay ensures that our practice remains solid and our commitment to a better life is strong.

Whether we've gone on a diet, set out to overcome an addiction, or simply want to change a bad habit, most of us can relate to abstaining from behaviors that don't serve us. Though this may seem like a difficult task, abstaining from certain things can have a powerful impact on our day-to-day lives. When we stop eating poorly or indulging our addictions, our entire lives open up to greater health and happiness. If we work to let go of behaviors that have a taxing effect on our bodies and minds, we naturally open ourselves up to behaviors that have an enriching influence. Patanjali proposes five behaviors to abstain from:

- VIOLENCE

- DISHONESTY

- STEALING

- SEXUAL EXCESS

- GREED

These five behaviors perpetuate the suffering of body and mind. When we exhibit violence toward others, we fill our minds with angry, hostile thoughts. When we are dishonest, we fill our minds with anxiety and fear about being called out on our falsehoods. Anger, fear, and other problematic emotions add to our burden in life, bringing on health issues, personal turmoil, and general unhappiness. The first ten weeks of the One Plan focus on the abstentions, and you will spend two weeks with each of these five behaviors, exploring how to eliminate it from your life.

The next set of behaviors encompasses those we want to incorporate into our lives. These are the observations. Patanjali teaches us to cultivate behaviors that enrich our state of being and help us be more centered. Incorporating these behaviors into our lives prepares us for higher practices like meditation. But even more important, the observations solidify our commitment to ourselves as being worth this effort; it's an exploration of self-affirmation. The five observations we'll pursue are

- PURITY

- CONTENTMENT

- AUSTERITY

- SELF-STUDY

- SELF-SURRENDER

As we did with the abstentions, we will spend two weeks exploring each observation, for a total of ten more weeks of the program.

The One Plan is based on the principle that we can enjoy the benefits of less suffering without taking on the whole of Patanjali's system all at once. These first twenty weeks will allow you to gradually incorporate the abstentions and observations into your life in the realms of the body, mind, or spirit. After pursuing these practices in the twenty weeks laid out for you, you will have built a foundation on which you may then construct a life of peace and fulfillment.

from darkness to light

NONVIOLENCE

I_T HAD BEEN A LONG TIME SINCE I HAD MET SOMEONE WITH A SMILE LIKE_ Somaly Mam's. She and I were on a small plane that would take us from Monterrey, Mexico, to Dallas/Fort Worth International Airport for our connecting flights. This hour-and-a-half flight came on the heels of another peace summit featuring His Holiness the Dalai Lama, where Somaly had been a speaker and I had led a meditation session in recognition of the tenth anniversary of 9/11.

Somaly's smile had a quality that I had seen before. Plenty of people have kind, warm smiles that suggest they have tremendous love to offer the world—especially people who are connected to the Dalai Lama's peace summits. But it wasn't until after we had landed in Dallas and were waiting for our connections that I realized why Somaly's smile looked so familiar. I had the opportunity to visit Nelson Mandela in 1998 during his time as president of South Africa. The house of Versace had invited me and a number of other models, including Kate Moss and Christy Turlington, to visit Mandela at his home as part of a fund-raiser to benefit Mandela's Children's Fund. From the moment I set eyes on him, Nelson Mandela captivated me. Even though he had been imprisoned for almost thirty years for speaking his mind, he committed himself to peace. He didn't seek vengeance against his captors but instead called for unity and freedom for all people in the country. When Mandela smiled, I understood what it was like to see forgiveness in action.

As we sat there in Dallas, I listened to Somaly tell her story. She was born into extreme poverty in early 1970s Cambodia. As the dangerous and destructive reign of the Khmer Rouge killed a fifth of the country's population, her family resorted to desperate means to survive. When she was still a child, she was sold as a slave to a man she had to address as "grandfather," and was abused by this man until she was sold to a brothel at the age of fourteen. She served multiple clients every day, was imprisoned in an infested cellar when she refused to allow her body to be used by a client, and was forced to marry a man who repeatedly beat and raped her. After watching a pimp murder her best friend, she escaped and, in 1993, fled Cambodia with the help of a French aid worker.

Then she went back.

In 1996, Somaly founded a nonprofit organization in Cambodia that seeks to rescue girls from brothels. In 2007, she founded the Somaly Mam Foundation in the United States, which likewise serves victims of sex trafficking. When Somaly realized that child prostitution was an enormous issue throughout the world, she set out to help the victims, and did so without any of the bitterness, rage, or other destructive feelings so often born from a painful childhood. When Somaly Mam smiled on that plane ride to Dallas, she not only showed love for those around her, as did so many people at the peace summit, but she showed love for everyone—including those who had imprisoned and tortured her for much of her life. She, like Mandela, smiled with the power of total forgiveness.

Somaly has found the strength in herself to let go of all her pain, and has used that strength to keep others from suffering the same fate. As of this writing, she has helped rescue over four thousand girls from sexual slavery.

Identifying Violence

Somaly dealt with extreme violence back in Cambodia. Though extreme physical violence may seem far from your everyday experience, violence takes place all the time and in many more ways than you might think.

Violence includes any action or thought that harms you or another. If we embrace this definition, do actions like gunplay and physical assault truly encompass all acts of violence? What about yelling at someone? Does that harm them? Does eating food that gives you high blood pressure harm you? Does a long-standing, deep-seated hatred for someone else make you feel good inside, or does it make you feel bad? When you see someone "being brought to justice," do you feel peaceful and warm, or do you fill yourself with righteous anger?

In the bigger picture of our lives, violence takes many forms. The world is filled with people who eat, drink, and smoke their way into the grave. It is filled with people flipping each other off for everything from being bumped into on the sidewalk to being cut off in a near car accident. Most of us have said hurtful things about other people behind their backs. And all of us have said hurtful things to ourselves.

All these actions—and many, many others—perpetuate pain. When we act from anger, we stir up anger in others. When we act from fear, we reflect the fear in others. When we consume substances that don't benefit our bodies, we harm ourselves. Each time we experience pain and then perpetuate that pain instead of resolving it or letting it go, we commit an act of violence.

In the first step of the Eightfold Path, Patanjali introduces *ahimsa*—the Yogic practice of nonviolence. When we participate in nonviolence, we choose not to perpetuate the pain of violent acts. We no longer flip people off for misunderstandings at a stop sign. We no longer burden our bodies with harmful substances. We no longer promote harmful thoughts in ourselves and others. Were each person to truly live in complete nonviolence, we would eliminate not only war and murder but disease and despair as well. People would resolve misunderstandings through productive acts of kindness and overcome conflict from a place of peace.

Is it any wonder that Patanjali placed this practice first?

From Darkness to Light

When she was able to feel love for her captors, Somaly Mam exhibited the highest form of nonviolence. However, between assaulting another human being and loving the person who assaulted you is a wide scale that defines our path from suffering in darkness to living with the spirit in light. In the first two weeks of the One Plan, I'll suggest ways to begin your practice of nonviolence in the realm of the body or continue with an existing practice of nonviolence in the realm of the mind or spirit.

The Body: Physical Nonviolence Toward Yourself and Others

Back in my modeling days, I had a disciplined workout ethic. I sought outer beauty so that I would be alluring to clients. But I also ate a lot of sweets, and at times I almost put myself into a diabetic coma. My teeth didn't fare well either. Though many actions can be labeled violent, the most basic and obvious way of inflicting harm is through the body. Yes, physically assaulting someone is a form of violence, for you are using your body to harm theirs. But filling yourself up with sweets is also a form of violence: it can lead to obesity, diabetes, and a host of other diseases that cause physical harm to our bodies.

Physical violence is any action that harms someone else's body or our own. This means that physical violence includes, along with physical assault and yelling, consciously doing things that compromise our health and well-being. Below are some behaviors that most of us consider a normal part of life but that actually do harm to our bodies.

WE EAT LATE AT NIGHT

A staple of modern life is eating late at night. We might have a snack of chips or cookies shortly before going to bed or a full-scale meal when everyone else is watching the opening monologue of a late-night comedian. But when we sleep, our bodies shut down and operate on the bare essentials. All systems of the body, like the circulatory and nervous systems, slow their activity while we sleep so that the body can regroup and commit energy to preparing itself for another day of functionality. The digestive system is no exception, as the digestive strength of the gastrointestinal tract greatly lessens so that the body can channel its strength toward activities like repairing cells.

It takes at least four or five hours for food to be fully digested in the stomach. When we eat before going to bed, we are burdening the digestive fire with matter it can't possibly burn off. It is like putting wet logs on a campfire: the logs won't burn until the next day, when they have dried out and the fire is relit. Food sits in the stomach and intestines and grows toxic overnight. It causes us to wake up feeling stiff, lethargic, and often with a sour taste coming up in unappealing burps. Because the body's systems are compromised as they try to get rid of this food, they no longer work together efficiently to sustain the body's immunity; thus people who eat late at night are more susceptible to illness like allergies and high cholesterol.

WE EAT PROCESSED AND GENETICALLY MODIFIED FOODS

Each of us is an organic being, and we are made from the same elements from which all of nature is made. However, our grocery stores are filled with processed foods that are nothing like the natural foods our bodies crave. When we consume synthetic substances, such as chemical preservatives or products that have been genetically modified, we're ingesting a toxic combination instead of a healthy one. When we consume something that doesn't come directly from the earth, we're putting into the body something it must get rid of—not something from which it can extract nourishment. We might as well swallow a plastic toy or imbibe windshield wiper fluid.

WE EAT FOODS FROM FAR AWAY

When we shop for produce at the supermarket, we often wind up buying tomatoes from Chile, bananas from Mexico, and other produce from who knows where. But when food is transported halfway around the world, it is harvested before it is fully ripe and then exposed to all sorts of toxins during transport. This compromises the nutritional value of the food. In contrast, foods from local farmers' markets are sold soon after being harvested, they are exposed to lower levels of toxicity, and they always reflect what is in season locally.

WE EAT MEAT

Most of the meat and fish sold in today's markets comes from farms using artificial growing practices and polluted water. The animals are fed corn instead of being allowed to graze naturally, and are often injected with hormones. These practices greatly reduce the nutritional value of the animal's flesh. Furthermore, foods like meat, poultry, pork, and other animal proteins are low in water content and difficult to digest. The more difficult foods are to digest, the more resources our bodies have to commit to processing them through the gastrointestinal tract. This leaves fewer resources for maintaining other systems, particularly the immune system. Thus eating a lot of meat is likely to make us sick more often.

WE EAT LARGE MEALS

Believe it or not, it is better to eat small amounts of unhealthy food than large amounts of healthy food. When we give the stomach too much to digest, it has to work overtime to process everything, much like it does when we consume dense foods, like meat. And just like with eating meat, this compromises the immune system as well and also causes us to be sick more often.

WE EAT SALADS

"What? Is that a typo?" you might be asking yourself right now. "How could Yogi Cameron be down on salads?" Western culture is obsessed with eating salad as a way to keep weight down. However, there is very little nutrition in foods like lettuce, and Ayurvedic tradition teaches that cooked foods are easier to digest than raw foods. When the food's fibers are broken down by cooking, processing the food requires less digestive fire. Since raw food is more difficult to digest, it puts a strain on the gastrointestinal tract, leading to indigestion and gas. Though people may develop particularly strong digestion over time and benefit from eating more raw foods, it is harmful to make such foods a staple of daily eating without a healthy digestive system.

WE EAT INCOMPATIBLE FOODS

There are many standard dishes in Western cuisine that aren't actually good for us, such as yogurt parfaits with berries or dry cereal with milk. Ayurvedic tradition teaches us to not mix certain kinds of foods, for foods have different enzymes and different properties. Eating them together can lead to gastrointestinal distress and accompanying symptoms (such as flatulence, acid reflux, diarrhea, or constipation). We shouldn't combine dairy with most fruits (but bananas are okay), nor should we combine dairy with animal protein, fish, or sour tastes like pickles. We shouldn't eat cooked foods and raw foods in the same meal. And we shouldn't eat dry foods with too much liquid. These combinations can hinder digestion and cause imbalance in the body. Also, it is important to not consume more than half a cup of warm water with a meal, because drinking too much liquid—especially when the liquid is cold—puts out the digestive fire.

WE EAT LEFTOVERS

Yes, I know. That tasty dish you brought home from the restaurant last night was *so yummy,* and having it for lunch today is a major step up from the cheese sandwich you would have had otherwise. And sometimes, it's just easier to prepare a big dish one night and then siphon it off for several days by zapping servings in the microwave for quick hot meals. Birthday cake can taste even better the day after the candles were blown out. But preparing food, storing it in the fridge, reheating it, and putting it back beats up the nutritional value of the food, sort of like a tennis ball that has been knocked back and forth on the court for too long. The food eventually loses its nutritional value, just as the ball loses its bounce. By the time the leftovers reach your stomach, they have as much nutritional value as cotton candy. When the body is given food with less nutritional substance, it needs more of it. When you eat more food, you gain weight. The violence toward the body continues from there.

Using the microwave to prepare frozen foods creates an unnatural and toxic environment for the food. And when frozen foods are cooked, frozen, and then cooked again, they lose their nutritional value. It is always better to cook natural, fresh food on the stovetop or in the oven.

WE DRINK ALCOHOL AND STIMULANTS

I know what you're thinking: alcohol, coffee, energy drinks, and sugary drinks like soda are staples of our lifestyle, so why would we *ever* say no to such tasty things? Drinking coffee, particularly first thing in the morning, is like giving the kidneys a hard slap. No part of the body should be treated that way. Sugary drinks—especially when they're made with high fructose corn syrup and carbonated water—are about as nutritional as notebook paper and far more toxic. And alcohol—well, we call drunk people "intoxicated" for a reason. We might as well fill our bodies with turpentine for all the poison we're putting into them when we drink beer, wine, or liquor. Drinking any of these is an act of physical violence.

Cigarettes are bad. Drugs are bad. Consuming either is about as physically violent as it gets. If you are to make a total commitment to this path and its promises, there's no room for cigarettes or drugs in your life.

It is, of course, also physically violent to have temper tantrums, scream and yell at other people, and even just say mean and insulting things. Any use of body or voice to do harm to ourselves or others is a form of physical violence. To practice physical nonviolence, you must renounce harmful foods and screaming matches in favor of more peaceful behaviors. You must learn to eat natural foods (such as fruits, vegetables, and grains) bought from local farmers' markets and avoid eating late at night. When you have a conflict with another person, you must resist the temptation to yell at that person or otherwise engage in meanness and cruelty. You must avoid using your body in a way that harms yourself or another.

Most people do things that are harmful to their bodies, so you will likely begin your practice of nonviolence in the physical realm.

The Mind: Mental Nonviolence Toward Yourself and Others

A client once contacted me after reading my first book, *The Guru in You*. Though she lived in the United States, she was originally from the Caribbean, and when she reached out to me she was struggling in her twenty-five-year marriage. When she and her husband first met, he pursued her to such a great degree that though she wasn't initially interested she ultimately gave in and married him. She was a very capable woman who made a lot of money traveling the world to market projects and products. But she never felt fulfilled in her work, because her husband belittled her to maintain control. When she expressed an idea, he would say that it was stupid. The next day, he would suddenly have a new idea—the very one she had the day before. She thought her ideas weren't very good, and he took advantage of this mind-set to make her think she needed him.

When she contacted me, she wanted my advice on how to move forward with her life. She knew she didn't want to continue on her current career path; she felt pulled toward developing a spiritual practice and doing something to benefit the planet. She also knew that she had no feelings for her husband and hadn't for a very long time. "I know I shouldn't be in this marriage," she said to me. "But what am I supposed to do?" She feared moving on. She thought her ideas weren't worth anything, and though she didn't love her husband, she didn't see how her life could take shape without him.

After a series of conversations about her worth as a person and further guidance and support in the form of practices similar to those found in the One Plan, she discovered for herself what she needed to do. She bought her husband out of their business so that he would be willing to divorce her. She's now free of him and living her life. She sends me periodic e-mails about how joyful her life is and how she's ridding herself of projects she no longer wants to be a part of. She's even become a source of guidance and support for her friends.

Do any of my client's struggles sound familiar to you? Have you ever felt bad because of something someone said to you, something you said to yourself, or some thought that made you feel like a lesser person than you were? Have you ever had a negative thought about someone else and thought less of them as a person? Are you even experiencing those kinds of thoughts right now? All of us have some sort of negative thoughts about others, and many of us struggle to see our own worth. As I've continued on my path, I've come to realize that there are many people in the world whose experience of fear, anger, or other unpleasant emotions has a crippling effect on their ability to live a life of purpose. My client was a capable woman with many great ideas, but because she thought so little of herself, she couldn't envision a life other than the one she had. She wasn't living the life she wanted because she exhibited mentally violent behaviors.

Mental violence is any thought that promotes anger, fear, hatred, separatism, competition, or other harmful feelings toward yourself or others. Having such thoughts harms the body and mind—no matter whom those thoughts are about. When we have dreams of pursuing certain careers but think we are inadequate, we often don't pursue anything of substance in our lives; we harm ourselves by fearing failure. When we dwell on what we've lost and consider ourselves victims, we fail to create abundance and joy in new ways; we harm ourselves by grieving over what we can't control. When we blame others for our unhappiness, gossip about others behind their backs, and think nasty things about other people, we perpetuate our pain rather than letting go of it; we harm ourselves by defining our lives through anger, hatred, and conflict. When we live our lives in mentally violent ways, we allow the mind to play tricks on us and tell us that we're bad or inadequate—just like my client told herself that she wasn't capable of living without her husband.

To practice mental nonviolence, you must work to overcome thoughts that stem from negative emotions like anger, fear, worry, sadness, and grief. This means letting go of nasty things people say and do to you, accepting loss as part of life, and working to overcome fear of the unknown.

What is perhaps most significant about the relationship between physical and mental nonviolence is that when we avoid physically violent acts, like following a poor diet and drinking alcohol, we feel better and therefore have fewer mentally violent thoughts.

The Spirit: The Highest Form of Nonviolence

Somaly Mam set out to help alleviate the suffering of young girls who had experiences similar to her own, but she came to consider even her captors with love and acceptance. Similarly, Nelson Mandela brought about unity and peace in using his years of unjust incarceration as the basis of a mission to serve all of humanity.

The highest form of nonviolence is embracing the truth that each of us has the potential and the right to free ourselves of suffering, as well as the capacity to avoid inflicting suffering on others. We recognize that though every person on this earth may be in some form of pain and many of these people may have acted on that pain in highly destructive ways, every person also has a completely perfect spirit that wants to give itself to the world for the benefit of all. We recognize that only our ego sees itself as separate from other egos, and thus violence is a product of the mind. When we make nonviolence our daily practice through the actions we take, we express it outwardly throughout our time on earth. When we succeed in creating this reality for ourselves, we let go of the ego's need for control, leave the darkness behind, and live in light.

The Plan

To incorporate nonviolence into your life using the One Plan, you will be called on to shift your lifestyle over the course of two weeks. The extent and intensity of this shift will depend on whether you need to work on physical nonviolence by such actions as reducing your intake of harmful foods, or if you already sustain a physically healthy existence and will instead focus on the mental and spiritual realms.

The Realm of the Body

Much of your nonviolence practice in the physical realm will be reforming how and when you eat. Eating late at night burdens your entire body. Consuming processed, unnatural, genetically modified, and nonorganic foods compromises your digestion and wreaks havoc on your immune system. You'll benefit most from a physical nonviolence practice if you eat right before going to bed; you frequently eat meat, processed foods, and leftovers; you consume alcohol or smoke cigarettes; or you frequently find yourself yelling or otherwise being physically abusive to other people.

WEEK 1: *Increase the amount of time between when you last eat and when you go to bed.* On Day 1, avoid eating during the last hour before bed, then add ten minutes each night until by Day 7 you avoid eating during the last two hours before bed.

WEEK 2: *Reduce your intake of toxic foods and substances by half.* Below is a list of food types and substances that reflect physically violent habits. Add up how much of each item you eat in any given week, and consume half as much for this week and all weeks thereafter. If you eat beef three times a week, have it only one or two times, or eat half as much per meal. If you go through two bottles of wine in a week, have only one. Replace these foods with vegetables, fruits, grains, nuts, seeds, legumes, dairy, and natural sweeteners (maple syrup or honey). Replace juices, soft drinks, and alcohol with water and herbal tea. See Appendix A for more information on diet.

- Meat (beef, pork, poultry, fish, lamb)

- Microwavable food (popcorn, ready-to-eat meals)

- Frozen food (waffles, ice cream, frozen dinners)

- Leftovers

- Processed snacks (chips, crackers, cookies)

- Processed desserts (cake, candy, pastries, chocolate)

- Processed foods with many unpronounceable ingredients

- Poorly combined foods (dairy with fruit or animal protein)

- Meals in a bag, sauces, dressings

- Juices (from concentrate, not freshly squeezed)

- Soft drinks (soda, lemonade, juice from concentrate)

- Alcohol

- Cigarettes

- Drugs

WEEKS 1 AND 2: *Use the Presence Practice described in part 2 for your physical nonviolence practice.* Below is a series of questions you are to ask yourself each morning after waking. When you ask yourself a question, such as "Do I call other people names?" consider all the times and situations in which you do this. If your answer is no, move on to the next question. But if you do, by the end of five minutes you should have explored the different ways you exhibit this kind of violence and resolved to no longer call people names. If there's a particular object of your name-calling, be sure to get in a conversation with that person by the end of the week so as to exercise this new behavior. If you call people names behind their backs, notice when your desire to do this emerges and then avoid doing so. Once you've addressed one question and found clarity regarding the situations in which you exhibit those behaviors, move on to the next. The questions to ask yourself are these:

- Do I call other people names?

- Do I yell at people?

- Do I use profanity to attack others?

- Do I tell people that I dislike them, hate them, or have contempt for them?

- Do I gossip about people behind their backs?

- Do I watch programs that degrade others?

- Do I say nasty things about other people behind their backs?

- Do I slam doors in people's faces?

- Do I threaten others, either verbally or physically?

- Do I put people down to make myself feel better?

- Do I physically attack others?

Though these first two weeks may not put you through a boot-camp-like workout regimen, it's definitely intense. It's usually not until after my clients have given their lifestyle an overhaul like this that they see what an enormous impact this work can have. In fact, though the One Plan was conceived as a program of long-term growth, if you follow these first two weeks of physical nonviolence exactly as I've laid them out, you will likely receive many of the benefits of those lightning-fast transformation programs: weight loss, greater energy, and a beginning of the end of annoying and even debilitating symptoms. You will feel lighter, healthier, and more engaged than you've probably felt in years. I hope you follow Weeks 1 and 2 of this program to the letter, so you can quickly see the benefits of the program as a whole.

The Realm of the Mind

Like I mentioned earlier, I ate a lot of sweets when I was young. Through my pursuit of the Yogic and Ayurvedic path, though, I gradually learned to stop consuming what I ultimately knew wasn't good for me. I decided a long time ago that eating sweets was a form of violence toward my body, and I resolved to give them up. I succeeded in not eating them for a couple of months, but then I entered another phase in which I started again. Then I'd stop. Then I'd start again. I went back and forth like this for years, but an interesting thing started to happen: the phases in which I didn't eat them became longer, and the phases in which I did became shorter. Eventually, I was able to train my mind to not even crave such things, and now I hardly ever eat sweets. You will benefit from a mental nonviolence practice after you've been consistent in scaling back the harmful substances you put into your body, so eliminating them outright won't be too large of a next step. Your mind will likely struggle to wrap itself around a behavior so far from what other people consider normal ("No chocolate? Like, *ever?*"), but when you are able to shift out of this habit, you will be the better for it. Follow this two-part plan for these two weeks and the weeks that follow.

WEEK 1: *Continue building your late-night eating practice.* Begin on Day 1 by refraining from eating during the last two and a half hours of the day, then add half an hour each night until Day 6, when you will avoid eating during the last five hours of the day. On Day 7 and every day thereafter, avoid eating after 7 P.M. regardless.

WEEK 2: *Eliminate harmful foods and substances from your diet.*

DAY 1: Eliminate meat.

DAY 2: Eliminate frozen foods, microwavable foods, and other processed foods.

DAY 3: Eliminate chips, cookies, crackers, and other processed snacks.

DAY 4: Eliminate processed desserts.

DAY 5: Eliminate soft drinks and coffee.

DAY 6: Eliminate alcohol.

DAY 7: Eliminate cigarettes.

WEEKS 1–2: *Refrain from mental violence toward yourself.* Each of us has felt fear when doing something that takes us out of our comfort zone. One act of mental violence toward yourself is telling yourself you can't do something because you don't think you'll be successful at it. The real lack of success is in not even trying. Spend five minutes first thing in the morning using the Presence Practice to ask yourself if you ever say, either to yourself or to someone else, that you're incapable of doing something. Ask yourself, "Do I say . . .

- that I can't do my job?"

- that I can't find a new job?"

- that I can't stand my coworkers?"

- that I'm no good at driving?"

- that I'll never be able to quit smoking?"

- that I can't stop eating?"

- that I can't keep myself organized?"

- that I can't sing, dance, or be funny?"

- that I can't speak in front of people?"

- that I can't let my guard down and allow someone to get close to me?"

- that I can't put myself out there and invite others to spend time with me?"

- that I can't strike up conversations at parties?"

- that I can't find someone to share my life with?"

- that I can't feel good about myself?"

Ask yourself one question in the morning, observe your answer, and if you find that you do say such things, resolve to become more aware of when you make that comment to yourself or to others in the future. When you've caught yourself saying one of these things or something similar, take note of it and make your task for the week to take a step toward doing what you said you can't do. If, for example, on Day 5 of Week 1, you catch yourself saying that you can't speak in front of people, then by Day 7 go and sign up for a one-day workshop that helps people overcome their fear of public speaking. The most important thing is to train yourself to understand that living in fear of what you can't control is not really living at all. Embrace this idea as an act of nonviolence toward yourself.

The Realm of the Spirit

When you experience peace and love for yourself and all living beings, you will be practicing nonviolence in the realm of the spirit. In this realm, you will be able to modify your life so that you are no longer working to the point of exhaustion, consuming an amount or type of food that will make you sick, or doing anything else that harms your body or mind. You will not engage in competitions at any level of the mind or body, nor will you recognize someone of a different color, gender, or sexuality as being different from yourself. You will embody the qualities demonstrated by Somaly Mam in the story shared earlier. You will regard perceived wrongs toward yourself or a loved one as an opportunity to feel love for the one who supposedly did the wrong.

If you feel you will benefit from working in this realm, spend these two weeks considering those you may have perceived as wrongdoers in the past (a former boyfriend/girlfriend/spouse, a former friend, a former colleague, a criminal offender linked to yourself or your family). Go through a list of people and one by one start to release them from your consciousness so you can both be free of your negative energy toward them. When you feel unconditional love for them and compassion for the way they have suffered in their lives, you are truly starting to live in nonviolence. Spend these two weeks finding ways to offer this love to others.

Emerging as a Masterpiece

In these two weeks, you will begin to see significant changes. If you are practicing in the realm of the body, you will feel lighter and healthier, and will likely have lost some weight. You will fit into a smaller dress size. An older pair of pants may fit you for the first time in years. You'll probably sleep better too.

If you are practicing in the realm of the mind, you will benefit from the total elimination of processed and unhealthy foods. You will feel lighter and attain greater focus in the activities with which you fill your day.

Putting It Together

At the end of each section of this program, I will provide a basic daily task list. As more tasks are added to the program, I will break them down into those that fulfill your daily routine (first do this, then do this) and those concepts and behaviors that you must remember to apply on an ongoing basis (continuing to practice mental nonviolence toward yourself, for instance). I have not included tasks from the realm of the body in the list for the realm of the mind, for it is implied that you've already incorporated those tasks into your lifestyle if you're working in the mental realm. You may also find that you will benefit from working with one practice (like nonviolence) in the realm of the body, but with a different practice (like truthfulness) in the realm of the mind; feel free to adapt the program to meet these needs as you see fit. And also, note that tasks related to the realm of the spirit have not been included here, as practicing in this realm is less of a regimen and takes shape once the first two realms have been practiced for many years.

In the first two weeks of the program, your practice will be relatively simple to manage. If you are practicing in the realm of the body, your daily practice over these two weeks will look like this:

- Spend five minutes in the morning on your Presence Practice, with a focus on avoiding abusive or violent behaviors.

- Gradually work toward not eating for two hours before your bedtime by the end of the first week.

- Spend the second week replacing half the unhealthy foods and other toxic items you consume with natural foods.

And remember . . .

- Find an opportunity to practice physical nonviolence during both Week 1 and Week 2.

If you are practicing in the realm of the mind, your daily practice over these two weeks will look like this:

- Spend five minutes in the morning on your Presence Practice, with a focus on avoiding mental violence toward yourself in the form of "I can't" statements.

- Gradually work toward not eating for the last five hours before you go to bed, and no later than 7 P.M. by the end of the first week.

- Spend the second week replacing all unhealthy foods and other toxic items with natural foods.

And remember . . .

- When you catch yourself making an "I can't" statement, by the end of each week take one small step toward achieving what you don't think you can do.

more than just cherry trees

TRUTHFULNESS

MANY CHILDREN IN AMERICA HAVE HEARD THE STORY OF GEORGE Washington and the cherry tree. Young George, all of six, came by a hatchet that he used to whack down his father's prized cherry tree. When the man confronted his son about the deed, the boy replied, "I can't tell a lie, Pa. I did cut it with my hatchet." Overwhelmed with pride, his father said, "Glad am I, George, that you killed my tree; for you have paid me for it a thousandfold. Such an act of heroism in my son is more worth than a thousand trees, though blossomed with silver, and their fruits of purest gold."

This story became very popular after it was reported by Parson Weems in his 1800 book *The Life of Washington.* It is often used to show the benefit of telling the truth, as being forthcoming about his destructive act earned the boy praise instead of reprimand—and particularly exultant praise at that. We should tell the truth, says the story, for that is the most noble of actions.

Two Flowers

This story reveals how Western cultures perceive truthful behavior: noble, pure, and heroic. If we lie and behave falsely, we are impure. We are cowards. These labels, whether filled with admiration or with contempt, are the product of our perceptions as individuals.

We each have had life experiences that shaped how we perceive actions. In the story about Washington, his father showers him with praise for telling the truth. He could have gotten mad about what his son did, but because his background and values had taken shape in a certain way over the course of his life—or because he was just in a really good mood that day—he decided that the confession demonstrated heroism. It wasn't George's actions that were heroic; it's just that on that particular day his father perceived them that way. If George had chopped down the tree but did his "I can't tell a lie, Pa" spiel while throwing the hatchet at a passing servant and impaling the poor man, would Papa Washington still have thought that his son's actions were purest gold? Probably not. In both situations, young George would have told the truth, but he would have earned praise for only one. If telling the truth is always noble and heroic, then it shouldn't matter what else he was doing at the time. How could something as culturally prized as telling the truth also be so fickle?

Patanjali teaches something different. The Yogic practice of truthfulness, called *asteya,* refers to abstention from falsehoods—either expressed to others or experienced within—in favor of that which is honest and correct. But what does "correct" mean?

Imagine a beautiful day in which you look out the window to see two flowers taking in the sun. They are both large blooms saturated with a pinkish-reddish color. As you observe these flowers, you notice that one of the two flowers is attracting hummingbirds, while the other is left completely alone. From afar, it doesn't look like there is any reason why one of the flowers is attracting fauna and the other one isn't. But when you go outside and inspect them more closely, you realize that one flower is real and the other is made of silk. Of course a fake flower isn't going to attract the birds, because it doesn't contain any nectar.

Though it's unlikely that someone would leave a fake flower amid real flowers outside your window, I presented the above scenario to make the point that certain occurrences happen in life because they are the natural order of things. Flowers attract fauna because that is the natural truth of a flower's existence;

without nectar, no hummingbirds would have any use for it. This is the natural order of how plants and animals exist.

Given that we as organic beings also fit into this natural order, nature has laid out a course of perfect truth for each of us to find within ourselves. This truth is defined by the same Creative Spirit that compels the world's plants and animals to behave as they do. Our dependence on technology and modern conveniences often prevents us from experiencing this reality. But we each have the opportunity to tune back in to the basic truth of any given situation so as to begin to reclaim the perfection afforded by our presence in this world.

In this sense, it doesn't matter how someone else responds to our truth—such as confessing to chopping down a tree—because it's not praise that motivates us, but rather the burden of knowing what happened and the fear that attaches to withholding that information. In part 2, I explained the Presence Practice using the example of someone who is not enjoying the time spent with a friend. That person behaves untruthfully, making up excuses about why he or she can't hang out. The practice of truthfulness would be either to scale back the role this person has in our lives or to recognize that we value what he or she brings to our lives and discover a way to have a genuinely good time. Before a truthfulness practice, we are burdened with what we know to be true: we don't enjoy our time with the other person. This reality isn't dictated by someone else's perception of the situation or by what someone else thinks should happen. It is dictated simply by what we know to be true. Just as the Spirit awards a hummingbird with nectar when it finds a genuine flower, it provides us with balance and peace when we tune in not to what our minds think ("I should spend time with this person because I don't want to hurt her feelings") but to what our spirit shows us ("It's just not meant to be"). This is living in truthfulness.

If we have a choice of speaking honestly or falsely, we speak honestly so as to maintain the lightness of sharing correct information. If we have a choice of following a path we have no interest in or seeking a path that helps us find fulfillment and purpose, we try to do the latter so as to be on the correct path for who we are and to no longer be victims of our own fear. When we forsake dishonesty, abstain from false thoughts, and pursue what is correct, we relieve ourselves of both a physical and a mental burden. We no longer encumber our bodies with the anxiety of deception, and we no longer create thoughts we have no use for. We speak, think, and act truthfully, not because we want to be perceived as noble or heroic but because this is how we make way for a more fulfilling life. This is how we attract hummingbirds with our nectar.

Paving the Way for a
More Fulfilling Life

The pursuit of the Yogic practice of truthfulness, like other practices in Patanjali's Eightfold Path, is pursued through the realms of the body, the mind, and the spirit. When we seek what is honest and correct in what we do, who we are, and how we relate to the world around us, we will view the world from a place of Spirit. We will live without fear. We will experience the fulfillment that comes when we pursue a life of greater peace and joy.

The Body: Truthfulness Opens Us Up

A funny twist on the George Washington story relates not to George but to his biographer Parson Weems. Today it is widely considered that the cherry tree story didn't actually happen. Through most of the nineteenth century, however, the story was a popular anecdote about America's first president; it wasn't until the end of the century that Weems's reporting was put to formal scrutiny. Weems didn't actually have any reliable sources on the events. He has also been accused of plagiarizing much of his material about Washington from fiction. One of the most famous stories about truthfulness was not actually true!

Whenever we use our bodies to deceive others, we commit an act of untruthfulness within the physical realm. We use our bodies untruthfully when we speak, write, or otherwise express an outright lie. We do so when we cheat in a game or engage in infidelity without our spouse's consent. We even behave untruthfully when we tell someone we're "fine" when we're anything but "fine." Any situation in which we express something we know to be untrue will eventually take its toll on the body, as the body absorbs the emotions of the mind. People who have long-term affairs or otherwise practice deceit on an ongoing basis often have a hard time sleeping. Sometimes their digestion weakens or they experience other health problems. When we lie about our age, we are allowing our fear of what others think to add to our burden. Anything that perpetuates fear also perpetuates suffering. Choosing to be truthful with others will free up the body to function at its best, as well as alleviating emotional heaviness.

The Mind: Truthfulness Unclutters Our Thoughts

In the late 1990s, a friend of mine decided to open a restaurant in Manhattan. She described it to me as the biggest restaurant in New York City. Because she had found success with several restaurants before, I decided to join in the venture. She asked me if I wanted to be her partner, and I accepted. I was planning to leave the fashion business anyway. Though I knew I didn't want to be a model anymore, I had no idea what to do instead. Rather than spending time exploring what I wanted for my life, I jumped at the opportunity to work with my friend.

The restaurant was enormous. It was made up of two and a half floors, each of which could accommodate two hundred diners. During the day, I sat in the office and called people, much like a party planner. I invited people to come by for lunch or dinner, showed off the beautiful space to company representatives, and helped them plan their next big event or annual soiree. I had friends and private VIP guests come down and taste the work of the master chef. But because it took so long for the wait staff to get from one end of the restaurant to the other, service was slow. It was nearly impossible to keep two hundred seats filled up at any one time, and managing the enormous number of patrons and staff members was an immensely difficult task. All of these factors added up to this being a stressful time.

I realized a little over a year into the partnership that I had accepted my friend's offer only because I couldn't think of anything better to do and I found the enormity of the project appealing. I thought I could make a lot of money and achieve the same success as a restaurateur that I had found as a model. The problem, however, was that I didn't like the sorts of challenges one faces as a restaurateur. I left the business in 2000.

It wasn't until I started my formal study of Yoga and Ayurveda a couple of years later that I realized how much I had been flailing around during this period. I was living a life that I wasn't meant to live, and it increasingly burdened my mind. I would complain to myself that I didn't want to do something, looking at obstacles as impediments instead of calls to action. Ultimately, these thoughts reflected the reality that I wasn't living truthfully.

Living a life that isn't true to our nature creates clutter in the mind, whether it's thoughts surrounding a dreaded task or disturbances over a nonbeneficial relationship. If we are in a job that we hate, how much time do we spend complaining about the job to others or fuming over tasks we don't want to perform?

We benefit from freeing ourselves of these thoughts, just as a ballerina benefits from keeping the dance studio free of clutter. If a ballerina had to be concerned with furniture and piles of stuff while she practiced her routines, she wouldn't be able to fully immerse herself in techniques or choreography. Similarly, when we live our lives in a way that isn't true to our nature, we create clutter in our minds that we then have to work around. Falsehoods engender extra thoughts and feelings that are of no use to us, and these extra thoughts and feelings are like toxins that get in the way of our health and peace.

It is therefore important to live a life that is truthful to who we are. If we changed to jobs that were more fulfilling, we would no longer fill our minds with all those burdensome thoughts. A relationship that stimulates spiritual growth serves both ourselves and the other person. We benefit from acknowledging emotions for what they are, recognizing what we care about, and reflecting on our past with accuracy. When we find a situation that serves who we are, we unclutter the mind and create clarity. Rather than thinking, "Oh, that feels too hard and I wish I didn't have to do it," we think, "Oh, that will be hard, and it's time to get to work."

The Spirit: Truthfulness Creates Peace

You will find total peace when you abstain from violence toward yourself and others and are able to love even the most seemingly offensive perpetrators of harmful acts. Similarly, when you avoid speaking falsehoods and live a life that is a totally honest reflection of who you are, you will live in complete joy. Rather than allowing your ego to impose what it thinks is true based on history or popular belief ("I should remain in a career that makes me a lot of money regardless of how little I enjoy it, for society rewards the affluent"), you will be at peace with your life. The practice of finding truth is based on the concept that, in a state of perfect peace, the natural truth of existence emerges through our thoughts, feelings, and actions without any resistance.

When this happens, we live without fear. We are able to experience life without any misgivings about what it will take to fulfill our purpose. We are able to see all people, animals, plants, and even human-made things as manifestations of the Spirit. When we find balance in our bodies and minds, we no longer perceive any one word or action as true or false—but rather allow our own spirit to be realized and exist in the perfect singular truth of creation. Each spirit is perfect, and when we embody this perfection, our existence reflects what is true.

The Plan

Whereas nonviolence practice featured a combination of dietary changes and behavioral modifications, truthfulness practice focuses entirely on modifying your behavior. You will abstain from falsehood in the realms of the body and mind before fully realizing the truth of the Creative Spirit.

The Realm of the Body

To explore the most material form of truthfulness, you must reflect on how you give voice physically to who you are and what you do. Your task for Weeks 3–4 is to spend five minutes each morning using the Presence Practice much like you did with your nonviolence practice. The following questions will help you isolate the various ways you act untruthfully toward others. Ask yourself:

- Do I engage in infidelity?

- Do I cheat (in games, competitions)?

- Do I tell small lies (such as saying you were somewhere you were not)?

- Do I lie about my age?

- Do I lie about the past (such as prior work experience)?

- Do I lie about the future (talking of plans you have no intention of pursuing)?

- Do I glaze over the truth through politeness (saying "I'm fine" when you're really not)?

- Do I glaze over the truth through fear (covering things up in a social situation to impress somebody)?

- Do I agree to make plans with someone in the future when I really have no intention of doing so?

- Do I agree to actual plans I have no intention of keeping?

When you answer yes to a question, use your Presence Practice to reflect on how you can adjust your behavior to start eliminating this practice from your life. Then, when you catch yourself acting falsely, reverse your behavior. If you're engaging in infidelity, that behavior will have to end if you are to remain on this path. For the more subtle forms of untruthfulness, you'll need to catch the untruth when you say it, and then remedy the issue through spoken honesty (change your résumé to reflect where you've actually worked, tell the other person—as nicely as possible—that you'd prefer not to make plans). As before, if a situation doesn't present itself naturally, create circumstances through which you can practice truthfulness.

The Realm of the Mind

You will benefit from practicing truthfulness in the realm of the mind if you manage your speech and actions to the point of not outwardly behaving dishonestly, but you still misrepresent who you are and what you want for yourself. Your work in the realm of the mind will be to consider your job, your relationships, and other aspects of your life to determine if they are truthful reflections of your nature. If you determine that they are not, shift your situation—and therefore your thoughts—so that your reaction to a false existence no longer takes up space in your mind. Your task for Weeks 3–4 is to spend your Presence Practice asking yourself the following questions:

- Am I in a friendship that I don't want to be in?

- Am I involved in a romantic relationship that is no longer fulfilling?

- Am I being dishonest about my intentions for a relationship?

- Do I have a job that I don't want to be in any longer?

- Am I pursuing an activity that I have no interest in but feel I should do?

- Do I pretend to feel worse or better than I actually am?

- Do I feel misunderstood, lost, or alone when there are people I care about who are available to help?

- Do I think things that I know to be untrue ?

- Do I tell myself I don't want something that I really do want?

- Do I pretend to not care about something I really do care about?

This practice challenges you to turn inward and be honest about who you are and what you want in life. When you find yourself thinking something untrue or putting yourself in a situation that you don't want to be in and don't have to be in, resolve to do something about it by the end of these two weeks. If you're invited to go out with friends and agree to go even if that's not what you want, back out and be okay with disappointing them. If you find that you really don't like your job, take a step toward changing that before these two weeks are up. No matter what, honor your commitment to this path by not letting falsehoods dominate your life. This will clear the way for more beneficial experiences and beings to come into your life.

The Realm of the Spirit

You will benefit from exploring truthfulness in this realm when you have set out a life for yourself that is a complete reflection of fearlessness. Your work enriches your life, as do your relationships. Though you certainly have off days, you understand your purpose when working through them. If you really live a life that can be described in this way, then it is time to begin exploring not just your truth but the universal truth that is oneness with the Creative Spirit.

For these two weeks, each time you encounter an object, consider not what you think it is, but its inherent truth separate from your perceptions or anyone else's. If you encounter an acorn on the ground, is it simply something without value that has fallen from a tree, or is it a source of food for a passing animal? As you explore your truthfulness practice in this realm during these two weeks and beyond, consider whether anything you've known up to this point is actually true, or if it is simply what you think is true. When you let go of your own thoughts, avoid assigning qualities to what you see, and allow things just to be, you will be in Spirit. You will be living the only truth there is.

Emerging as a Masterpiece

Moving into Weeks 3–4, you will maintain your nonviolence practice but change the focus of your Presence Practice to truthfulness. Continue your eating habits from the first two weeks of the program. By now, you should have lost noticeable physical and mental weight and likely have more energy than you did. Ask yourself if you're finding the program to be manageable, or if the guidelines are starting to feel like restrictions. Given its less tangible nature, is truthfulness going to be harder for you to remain committed to? Are you finding more false words and thoughts than you anticipated? Do you feel impatient or empowered? Remember that this program is ambitious for anyone. But it also carries significant rewards for those who follow through.

Putting It Together

If you are practicing in the realm of the body, your daily practice over these two weeks will now look like this:

- Spend five minutes in the morning on your Presence Practice with a focus on refraining from speaking and behaving dishonestly. Refer to the list of questions as needed. Act on reversing at least one falsehood by the end of each week.

And remember . . .

- Continue eating half as much processed food and unhealthy substances as you did prior to the program. Avoid eating during the last two hours of the day.

- Continue building nonviolence behaviors to the best of your ability.

If you are practicing in the realm of the mind, your daily practice will look like this:

- Spend five minutes in the morning on your Presence Practice, with a focus on avoiding thoughts that reflect a lack of truth about who you are and what you want for yourself. Take a first step toward resolving a falsehood in your situation by the end of these two weeks.

And remember . . .

- Continue eating natural foods, and refrain from eating in the last five hours of the day or after 7 P.M.

- Continue catching your "I can't" statements.

the karma diet

NONSTEALING

T'S BEEN AT LEAST FIFTEEN MINUTES SINCE YOU ENTERED THE PARKING LOT, but here you are, still looking for a parking spot because the only time you could come to the store was right at the end of your workday. You just need a few things for a special dinner for some friends tonight, and now you can't find a spot because everyone's running last-minute errands. As the minutes go by, you realize you're close to not having enough time to prepare the meal.

You crane your neck to look for spaces. As you turn forward again, you suddenly see someone halfway out of a spot only two spaces from where you are. You close the small gap, turn on your signal, and swoop in with delight at having gotten a space, and right near the store's entrance.

Then the trouble begins. A man accuses you of taking his spot, insisting that he was waiting there with his signal on before you even knew it was there. You turn on him in defiance, and with a haughty edge to your voice, you ask him if he expects you to move. He tells you to forget it, grumbles under his breath, and drives on.

You continue on your very short walk to the store, pleased that you got your way. You did give him the opportunity to tell you to move, and he gave you the go-ahead to keep the spot. You can't help it if it takes him another ten minutes to make it into the store. That's his problem.

The Burden of a Super Value Meal

People in the West are prone to label actions right or wrong. Most people agree that stealing—taking something that isn't theirs—is wrong. We must punish those who steal, because they did something bad, and punishing bad actions is the right thing to do. It is justice.

As we explored over the last two weeks, eliminating falsehoods from our lives isn't noble, but it helps us stop afflicting our lives with more issues. Similarly, we don't avoid stealing because it is wrong but rather because it adds to our personal burdens.

Take the example of the parking space. Did you do anything illegal? No, of course not. But did your actions have ramifications? Yes, because the other person had to endure the inconvenience of not getting the space they had seen first. Though you may have suddenly become rather unpopular, it's not even the ill will that is of greatest significance. So why is it problematic to have acted that way?

To answer this question, I'd like you to imagine someone you might see in the food court of a mall. As you walk through the mall one day, you come across a man sitting by himself in the corner of the food court gorging on an extra-large value meal. You probably don't think this man is committing an immoral act or deserves justice. In fact, he might deserve a bit of sympathy. Not only is he eating unhealthy food, but he probably looks unhealthy because this is his regular eating habit. If he's harming anything, it's his digestive system. But, unhealthy or not, you probably agree that eating that way is his right.

Asteya, the Yogic practice of nonstealing, calls on us to avoid stealing because it will serve us, just as no longer eating fast food serves us. Our ego wants to control its surroundings, and taking something that isn't ours is simply the ego exerting its will. Stealing is an indulgence of the ego's need for control, and the only thing we gain by gratifying our ego is more suffering. But when we practice nonstealing, we undermine the ego's control. Doing so helps us be the lightest, most balanced person we can become. In the story about the parking space, the other person might very well have beat you to the spot while you were craning your neck looking for other spaces; by being so defiant and taking the space despite the likelihood that it was someone else's, your ego created a heaviness that you then have to contend with as your karma.

The law of karma states that every action has an opposite and equal reaction. A man who steals from a store's cash register must contend with the reality that someday his life will be defined by this action. Perhaps the thief will have something taken from him. Perhaps he continues to rob stores, and the work he does to conceal his thievery takes so much out of him that he has a heart attack and dies young. The owner of the store may seem like the only victim, but the thief has burdened himself with karma. If we assign a value of *bad* or *wrong* to the thief, we're making an unproductive observation. Instead, those of us on the Yogic path observe that a man who steals from a store must one day address that burden when he encounters the suffering that is his due. Were he to go on a karma diet and avoid stealing, he would shed that excess weight, so to speak.

We burden ourselves when we knowingly take something that belongs to someone else, such as a parking space, a purse, or even two hours of that person's life. We suffer because we used that person with the intention of getting what we wanted. You might argue that the thief doesn't care that he stole from someone else ("He has no moral center, Yogi Cameron!"), but all you need to do is to look at the high-powered CEOs involved in corporate scandals who die of heart attacks or other illnesses to know how much they burdened their health with their thievery.

There are, of course, some actions we may feel justified in taking because they have been deemed legal by our government. Just because it's legal, however, doesn't mean that it isn't a form of stealing and not bound by the laws of karma. Consider the large corporations that make sugary drinks and compromise their customers' health. They're stealing their customers' well-being. If you're like me, you've read many news articles or seen movies about the casualties of war. You may have even been to war yourself. Even though war may be formally declared, even though a soldier is following orders, he or she is stealing another person's life. We even steal from each other when we go on a date, size the person up, and rather than enjoying the company of a fellow human being, we tick off a checklist of expectations to see if they will fulfill our needs. When we spend time with someone but focus only on whether they measure up to our expectations, we're doing little more than using them and stealing their time as we move in to take what we want. Whether these actions are taken on behalf of profit, justice, or the search for love, they all have karmic ramifications.

Weeks 5–6 of the One Plan focus on the practice of nonstealing. The purpose of this part of the plan is to help you let go of behaviors that would otherwise burden you with poorer health, darker moods, and an unpleasant life. Step by step, we're chipping away at these habits to reveal the masterpiece within.

How Do We Avoid Stealing?

To avoid stealing, we must avoid taking from others. This is an absurdly simple statement, but we can only turn stealing into nonstealing if we are able to live this as part of our lives on a day-to-day basis. We practice nonstealing whenever we are presented with an opportunity to take what isn't ours but avoid doing so. When we pursue this through the physical, mental, and spiritual realms, we create a life free of karmic burdens.

The Body: Stealing Objects and Spaces

Stealing in the physical realm is defined as taking other people's physical possessions and physical space. This can involve taking valuables, money, or food. It includes stealing office supplies from our employers, cheating on our taxes, and of course stealing a parking space. It can even include stealing from the planet in the form of ecologically harmful habits. In each instance, we're acquiring something that exists in the physical world even though the situation dictated that it was to be possessed or shared by someone else. Physical nonstealing thus means refraining from using our bodies to steal physical items, monies, nature, and spaces from others.

The Mind: Stealing Other People's Time and Attention

I once worked with a client who experienced severe allergies and sought my services so that she could feel better. I had an initial consultation with her, where I asked her questions, took her pulse, and conducted other diagnostics. During the session, I taught her postures and breathing techniques, explained what herbs to take, and showed her lifestyle modifications she could make. She agreed to make these adjustments, and we set a time for me to come back the following week. When I came back to work with her again, she hadn't done any of the work I had prescribed. I asked her why she hadn't done anything, and she confessed that she thought I was going to take her through everything she was supposed to do—that I would be doing the work for her. I then asked her why she asked me to come a second time if she had decided not to participate, and she said she was still hoping that there was something I could do for her.

It is completely understandable that this woman might not have grasped the nature of the therapeutics I employ with my clients before I came to see her, but I certainly made the process clear during the consultation. Though she understood what she was expected to do, she chose not to do it. This was, of course, her choice, but knowing that she wasn't interested in doing what I prescribed to her but still having me come back again meant she was stealing my time, energy, and attention.

Whether we talk regardless of whether our companion is interested, create drama for the sake of attention, or otherwise take another person's time for granted, all of us have used our minds to steal from others. When we take someone's time without serving the other person in any way, we're using the mind to steal. This happens because this particular form of thievery is defined by imbalances of the ego.

When we talk to someone just to hear ourselves speak, or to start an argument, or to try to get something out of them like my client did with me, or otherwise only to serve ourselves, we're allowing the controlling dictator that is the ego to direct our behavior. We allow that dictator to steal our own well-being from those we care about when we take unnecessary risks like with base jumping and race car driving, and to steal other people's time when we burden them with our pain as a result of not living our purpose. In the ego's need for control, it tells us that we are only important if other people pay attention to us, that we must win an argument for our opinion to be validated, and that other people are only worth talking to if they can help us. None of these outcomes provides happiness. And yet the ego vies for control all the same, always wanting more. When we take up other people's precious time with the burdens of our ego, we're allowing our suffering to influence their experiences. We're allowing our suffering to stand in the way of their finding peace for themselves.

Our practice here is to avoid stealing other people's time by not allowing our ego to create situations that aren't of use to others. If we no longer steal people's time, we will no longer bog ourselves down with the weight of the ego's insatiable appetite for control. When we converse with someone who is suffering from their ego's desire for control ("And then this happened to me, and then that happened to me, and then they said to me . . ."), we can be present to their struggle by observing their need for attention. Perhaps, by being present to them, we can help them see how much they are dominating the conversation and help them let go of that need for control—though this doesn't happen often. However, if you help them make this discovery for themselves, then you have helped them alleviate some of their suffering. You have practiced compassion.

The Spirit: Give to Those Who Steal from You

You might know the story of Jean Valjean, the hero of Victor Hugo's novel *Les Misérables*. Shortly after being released on parole, Valjean struggles to find shelter, since no innkeeper will take in an ex-convict. He is eventually welcomed by Myriel, the bishop of Digne, and given a place to stay. During the night, Valjean runs off with much of the bishop's silver, only to be brought back by the police. But Myriel doesn't turn Valjean in. "I gave you the candlesticks too," he says in front of the policemen, "for which you can certainly get two hundred francs. Why did you not carry them away with your forks and spoons?" After the police leave, Myriel advises Valjean to use the silver to start a new life of honesty and godliness.

Your work in the spiritual realm of nonstealing is to fill your heart with love for all living beings, so if someone steals your wallet, you also give him your cell phone. When people steal your place in line at the movie theater, you buy a ticket for them. When you see people who steal from you not through their actions but through the perfection of their souls, you will also realize the perfection of your own soul. You will understand that every interaction with a thief is another opportunity to undermine the ego's control and serve the Creative Spirit. Just like Myriel gives even more to Valjean, so too will you give to all regardless—and because—of what they take from you.

The Plan

The practice of nonstealing in the One Plan relies entirely on use of the Presence Practice. Nonstealing, like truthfulness, is less a specific set of exercises and more a modification of behavior: we remind ourselves to not steal until we no longer do so. When we do remember not to steal and follow through on this practice, we achieve not just the lightness born of fewer burdens, but greater fortune and abundance.

The Realm of the Body

Though a nonstealing practice at the physical level includes not taking a pack of gum from the local convenience store, it also includes not taking a parking space claimed by another person or appropriating office supplies from your company's supply room for personal use. Even if it seems like it won't hurt anyone, it's still adding to your burden and your karma. You will benefit from practicing non-stealing in the realm of the body if you find yourself taking objects or spaces in even seemingly harmless ways. Spend five minutes of your morning routine using the Presence Practice to ask yourself the following questions:

- Do I ever shoplift?

- Do I ever take someone else's possession without their consent?

- Do I ever take free condiments and other fixings from a restaurant?

- Do I ever take more paper napkins than necessary?

- Do I ever cheat on the number of hours on my time sheet?

- Do I ever cut in line?

- Do I ever swoop in front of somebody as they're about to get in line?

- Do I ever cut someone off in traffic?

- Do I ever get onto a subway or train by holding open the doors while they're closing?

- Do I ever take a parking space someone else was waiting for?

- Do I ever not tell a cashier that they didn't ring up an item I am purchasing or that they gave me incorrect change in my favor?

- Do I ever use an item of clothing or some other item that I purchased with the intention of returning it?

- Do I ever read books at the bookstore and then put them back on the shelf without buying them?

- Do I acquire pirated software, music, or video content?

- Do I ever use company supplies for personal use?

- Do I ever use company technology, personnel, or other components for personal use?

- Do I ever wait until a parking enforcement official is about to write a ticket before feeding the meter?

- Do I ever lie on forms to pay fewer taxes?

- Do I ever lie about age to get lower admission at movie theaters and other venues?

- Do I ever create large amounts of waste instead of recycling?

- Do I ever use gas-guzzling cars and other pollutants instead of more fuel-efficient options?

When you find yourself about to commit any of these acts, simply stop, do what you need to do to rectify the situation (give back the extra money to the cashier, allow the other person to take the space), and continue on with your day. If you haven't been in a situation to avoid stealing by the end of Weeks 5 and 6, put yourself in a position to do so (such as investing in a monthly TV Internet streaming service instead of watching free pirated content). Consider reading through this list of actions at the beginning of your five minutes to remind yourself of the behaviors you're looking to avoid.

The Realm of the Mind

If you are stealing physical objects and spaces, it will be all the more difficult to avoid mental types of stealing—like having one-sided conversations or creating drama for the sake of attention. How can we see the value in avoiding conversations that have no value to others if we're still pocketing that twenty dollar bill the cashier mistakenly gave us or taking that stack of Post-its from the office to use at home? You will benefit from practicing nonstealing in the realm of the mind after you have succeeded in abstaining from material forms of stealing. To practice nonstealing at the mental level, use the Presence Practice to ask yourself the following questions:

- Do I have conversations with others that are only about myself?

- Do I use conversations with others as a way to gratify my ego instead of serving their interests?

- Do I talk only about subjects that are of interest to myself?

- Do I smother a child for the sake of getting more attention?

- Do I use other people just to have sex even if they want a more emotionally significant experience from me?

- Do I demand attention while people are trying to do something else?

- Do I perform in front of people to get money out of them instead of purely to entertain them?

- Do I explain things to others in a boring and uninspired way instead of in an understandable and caring manner?

- Do I constantly play martyr or victim at the expense of another person's needs?

- Do I take up additional time in customer service environments to complain about my situation without any intention of resolving the issue?

- Do I take up other people's time by complaining about things I have no plan to change?

- Do I create drama to get attention?

- Do I maintain a friendship without a genuine interest in spending time with the other person?

- Do I spend time at work conducting personal activity?

- Do I spend time at work chatting with coworkers instead of working?

- Do I seek or give favor within government agencies through personal contacts?

- Do I find loopholes in an official system for personal advantage?

- Do I befriend people not because I want to be their friend but because I want to date them?

One client came to me because of ringing in his ears. He complained to his partner about it all of the time. After we started to work together and his symptoms dissipated, he realized how difficult he was making his partner's life and in turn his own. Instead, he began to focus on how he could serve his partner's needs. His ailment subsided, and his relationship became more positive.

In constantly complaining about his ailments, my client was stealing his partner's time. When you realize you're having thoughts that cause you to steal other people's time and attention, simply stop yourself. Avoid sticking your hand in the closing subway doors or engaging someone in a conversation because you want attention. Over these two weeks, you'll begin to see how often opportunities to steal creep into your life. When you choose not to, you'll be the lighter for it.

The Realm of the Spirit

When you find yourself engaging others so that you may enrich their lives, and you avoid taking even the smallest bit of time to serve yourself at the expense of others, you will be ready to serve the Creative Spirit. Rather than look for an opportunity to give, you allow situations in which you may practice to present themselves to you naturally and continuously.

Your practice for these two weeks is to prepare to give to those who steal from you and others. Rather than seeing this as enabling their supposed wrongdoing, conduct yourself as Bishop Myriel did in *Les Misérables* and wish that they may move away from perpetuating their own personal hell. Here, when the rest of the world offers that person only scorn and vengeance, you will offer them your love—and your wallet.

Emerging as a Masterpiece

A month into the program, you will not only feel lighter in the stomach, but you should also feel lighter in the mind. Some of the largest chunks of marble are getting knocked off, and the results of your work will start to become more subtle. As you continue to build on these new behaviors through these two weeks of nonstealing, the behavioral modifications you've already made in the first four weeks of the program will likely start to be replaced by old habits; you will sometimes feel like you're not on a program of spiritual growth at all. But when you keep at it, it will become a part of your lifestyle. Just keep reflecting on the habits you want to move toward. As you chip away and become more aware of your behaviors, the benefits of this lifestyle will fall into place.

Putting It Together

If you are practicing in the realm of the body, your daily practice over these two weeks will now look like this:

- Spend five minutes in the morning on your Presence Practice, with a focus on refraining from stealing physical objects and spaces. Remember to place yourself in a situation to practice this behavior by the end of the week if the opportunity doesn't present itself naturally.

And remember . . .

- Continue eating half as much processed food and unhealthy substances as you did prior to the program, and avoid eating during the last two hours of the day.

- Continue building your nonviolence and truthfulness behaviors to the best of your ability.

If you are practicing in the realm of the mind, your daily practice over these two weeks will look like this:

- Spend five minutes in the morning on your Presence Practice, with a focus on refraining from stealing through conversations, subpar work, or other thievery of the mind. Place yourself in a situation in which to practice at least once by the end of each week.

And remember . . .

- Continue eating natural foods. Avoid eating in the last five hours of the day and after 7 P.M.

- Continue your nonviolence and truthfulness practices.

- Continue to mix and match the different realms of your practice if you find yourself more within the physical realm of one area but in the mental realm of another.

the tricky one

CONTINENCE

TRIED TO BE CELIBATE IN MY LATE TWENTIES. IT SEEMED LIKE A GOOD IDEA at the time. I had had a series of committed relationships throughout my early and mid-twenties, including being married for a little over a year. The last of these relationships lacked any seriousness or purpose, so on the advice of my mentor, I broke it off and went solo for a few years. During this time I didn't have any sex. Well, at least not with anyone else. Though I considered myself celibate because I wasn't having any contact with anyone, I was still finding release through thoughts, imagination, and . . . the obvious. After this spell of being alone, I embarked on a relationship that lasted nearly ten years. It was the most beautiful relationship I could have imagined.

Eventually, we ended the romantic aspects of our relationship because we both wanted to explore a higher path on our respective journeys. I travel to India every year to further my education and practice with my guru, and I did this shortly after our relationship ended. Over the years, my guru had taught me that refraining from releasing one's sexual essence promotes health and longevity, as well as allowing one to focus on living a more purposeful and joyful life. According to him and Yogic texts in general, this essence is the most powerful force in body and mind, and it should be reserved for spiritual purposes. Given that I had just ended a lengthy and emotionally significant relationship, I looked at my India trip as an opportunity to consider a more authentic celibacy: this time I would avoid any release, either physical, mental, or emotional. Perhaps my travels helped me focus on the work I was doing, but celibacy wasn't as much of an effort as it had been when I was younger. By this point, I was far more grounded in my practice—or so I thought.

Rural India is a wonderful place for being still and grounded. It allows you to be alone and surrounded by others of like mind. But back in the West, the energy is one of sexual contention. When I returned to the States, I got involved with someone, and it was primarily a sexual experience. Initially, I tried to stay focused on my work. I received a lot of attention from this woman, but I allowed it to come without feeling the need to respond. However, I soon began to feel a lustful attachment. It became a distraction. I let my guard down and experienced sexual tension as a result. If I had been looking for a relationship, this would have been one of those wonderful and beautiful times in life when everything seems perfect. But I knew I needed to focus on my practice and work. I didn't want to be distracted by anyone or anything. Even though it wasn't something I wanted or sought out, I wound up succumbing to the sexual allure of the situation. I experienced two contrasting mind-sets at once: I wanted to remain focused on my path, but I also wanted this woman. I may have thought I was grounded in my practice and my purpose, but it turned out that my willpower just wasn't strong enough. I made the grave mistake of underestimating the power of sexual energy. My guru teaches that sexual energy is a source of calm, creativity, and bliss when it is under control, but because it was out of control it became wild and destructive.

After several months, I managed to detach from what was turning into an unhealthy situation for both of us. It took all my strength and every ounce of discipline I had created through my practice to do it, but I managed to disassociate from the control this sexual energy had over me. If there was ever an indication of how much power could be gained from my sexual potency, this was it: never before had I had to work so hard to achieve something in my practice as when I resumed celibacy. In turning my spiritual practice into action, I was shown its strength.

Our Most Creative Act

I know what you're thinking. "Why, Yogi Cameron, are you about to teach me about sexual abstinence?" Or, when reading the above story, you may have thought, "If someone was giving you sexual attention, you're both consenting adults, and the sex is enjoyable, and the sex is enjoyable, and the sex is enjoyable, why is it hurting anyone? Isn't that the sort of thing most of us are searching for?"

When Patanjali describes continence in the Yoga Sutras, he says that avoiding sexual release leads to strength, vigor, vitality, and courage. And in true Yoga Sutra style, he says little else on the subject. Each sutra is concise, a simple strand of truth, and he leaves it to us to integrate this information into our practices and lives according to where we are on our path. If we skipped over it in our practice, we would be bypassing a valuable tool for creating a life of fulfillment and peace. How can abstaining from something so enjoyable lead to peace? This is why *brahmacharya,* Yogic continence, is "the tricky one."

We are mentally programmed to enjoy the sexual act because—at least traditionally—this is the only way to propagate the species. If sex didn't lead to pleasurable sensations, human beings would have been far less likely to procreate, and the species might have died out long ago. But continence isn't about abstaining from procreation; it simply helps us become more aware of when to bring another spirit into the world. When we have sex for the sake of having sex, we gratify our senses and experience pleasure. But when we have sex for the sake of procreation, we conceive a child in a balanced state. This balance then manifests itself in how the child comes into and exists in the world.

Why should sexual moderation even be worth talking about, let alone be included in this ancient system? The most significant creative act is the creation of a new life, and this makes sexual essence our most potent substance. The body has to rally all its resources to produce it, and repeatedly depleting this essence leaves the body with greatly reduced resources to keep the immune system intact or sustain the body's vitality, for instance. Repeatedly releasing your sexual essence is like draining a plant of moisture—what is left is a sickly, dried-out organism. Even if it manages to stay alive, it never looks or feels as good as it once did.

In many Western cultures, a stigma is attached to people who have a lot of sex—particularly women, and especially those who have a lot of sex with multiple partners. Just like the act of stealing we explored in Weeks 5–6, the Yogic path doesn't stigmatize having a lot of sex but rather shows us that partaking in such activity is bad for our health and peace—even if it is sex with the same partner. Rather than a moral issue, it's a physical, mental, and spiritual one.

As you know, we obtain energy from the food we eat. Our digestive systems metabolize that energy, which our bodies use to maintain bodily systems. Ayurveda teaches us that when we consume food, our bodies distribute the energy into seven levels of tissue. First, the energy becomes plasma. Then it becomes blood. From there it becomes muscle, fat, bone, and marrow. After the energy has become marrow, it is finally ready to become reproductive tissue (semen or ovum). Each phase is created from the previous phase, so the reproductive seed must pass through the most transformations. Barley and grapes lack any potency in their original form, but when they're fermented into beer and wine, they become far more potent. Similarly, the body must invest significant resources to create the sexual seed as a force potent enough to create life; it is only the most refined energy that can help us create another being. In a manner of speaking, this seed is the most fermented of bodily tissues. This gives reproductive tissue tremendous creative power, and depleting it saps the body of the results of this extensive process.

The energy that goes from food all the way to reproductive tissue is known in Ayurvedic teachings as *ojas*. Given that the sexual seed is the essence of all creation in the body, releasing it requires the body to rally a large amount of *ojas* to restore and replace it. And the more work the body has to do to replace the seed, the less *ojas* it has to sustain the rest of the body—including the immune system.

But though it is easy enough to see how sexual release can undermine our physical health, how might it undermine our peace? As the energy responsible for all human life, it affects all aspects of our existence. On any given day, a person who has an active interest in sex will relate to the world around as a possible outlet for release. Though they might not act on it by pursuing others, their desire affects how they conduct themselves in any given moment. It influences how a conversation might go, what sort of impression one might have of another, and ultimately, how a relationship might develop with another person. Imagine if a man met a woman whom he desired in a sexual way. Without acting on his interest, he forms a friendship with her that he describes as platonic but secretly wishes were otherwise. He then grows frustrated and even angry that he isn't getting his way. Indeed, the creative force contained in sexual desire is so strong that when someone completely loses control of it, their frustration and anger can turn into rage; this is how someone with deep-seated frustrations can eventually become a molester or rapist.

Our sexual energy can be destructive and wasteful when we use it to simply have sex, but it can also be immensely healing and life changing when we reserve it for soul searching. When this power is used for pursuing projects, a career, or even serving others in a selfless capacity, it can be more powerful than the highest political office. My struggles with the sexual relationship I described above demonstrate that this practice is by no means easy to attain. But the pursuit of continence underlines why one must commit to a spiritual practice on a daily basis for a lifetime: we never know when we will be tested and need to draw on the strength and discipline we find through this work. Sri Ramakrishna Paramahamsa said, "A man practicing brahmacharya for twelve years develops a special power. Special power to know and understand everything seen and unseen. He gets to know God." When we succeed in finding the discipline to attain sexual moderation or abstention, our sexual energy will shift the world around us—but also our world within.

The Promises of Moderation

Through the three realms of existence, the practice of continence manifests in two phases: moderating sexual activity, and channeling the reserved energy into heightened creativity. There are many ways to explore this process.

The Body: Continence Creates Vigor

I once worked with a client who suffered from severe acid reflux disease. I prescribed scaling back the sex he had with his wife, for they had a particularly active sex life. Though this is something many couples may envy, the constant heating up of the body—as well as the depleting nature of his sexual release—was affecting the severity of his symptoms. The muscles are especially affected by too much sex, and damage leads to deep fatigue, hair loss, loss of sight, migraines, impaired hearing, and other indications of wasting away. This is why we are tired after sexual exertion. You might have also noticed that some people have more vigor than others and can experience greater sexual release without getting tired. One person may be tired after only releasing this energy one time, while another person may be able to repeat three or four times over several hours. If we feel fine after release, then we have a greater reserve of *ojas*. But no matter what, there is a point of depletion for each person. When we retain our sexual essence in the body, we create and maintain greater strength and energy. Continence requires us to refrain from sexual release at least enough to avoid fatigue. When we succeed in doing this, we will experience greater vigor.

In the physical realm, continence is the practice of preserving one's sexual energy and using it for creative endeavors. To do this, we have less sex, we gratify ourselves less, and we don't seek out situations in which we try to have sex for the sake of it. We avoid exposing ourselves to pornographic content, as well as other images, songs, or stimulation that is sexual in nature. Putting this much attention on pursuing sexual gratification increases the draining qualities of sex, as we're investing energy and time into the pursuit itself. Even the person who goes to a bar and strikes out, experiencing no sexual release at all, has still committed his or her body to the pursuit of sex. To practice continence in the realm of the body, you must reduce both sexual release and your focus on finding a sexual partner.

The Mind: Continence Improves Productivity

If continence in the realm of the body centers on abstention from the physical pursuit of sex and sexual release, then it should be no surprise to you that continence in the realm of the mind centers on abstaining from thoughts about sex. Though it may be challenging to abstain from physical actions, it is certainly straightforward. Either we're having sex, seeking sex, and watching things related to sex, or we're not. But abstaining from thinking about sex is more ambitious. If we're constantly wishing for sexual release, we are compromising our mental health. If we send out vibes about people's sexually appealing attributes ("Wow, nice ass"), or are constantly thinking, "I really wish I were having sex right now," we wind up relating to people as objects of desire. These actions may not deplete the body, but they dull the mind and lead to frustrations or imbalances in our thoughts. They will eventually lead to sex or to frustration for not having it, or they will land us in trouble as we chase our desires. And most significantly, they will distract us from thinking about more productive things.

When we train ourselves to avoid frequent sexual thoughts, we make way for more productive actions. These actions will in turn encourage more loving and unified moments with everyone. Rather than thinking, "I wish I were having sex," we might think of a new and interesting way to solve a problem at work. We might have a brilliant new idea for a project we would like to start, and because we're no longer draining ourselves, we'll have the energy to pursue it. Just like eliminating untruthful thoughts clears the way for truthful ones, eliminating sexual thoughts clears the way for creativity to flow. These productive, creative thoughts do not originate from a place of desire, so they no longer lead to selfishness. In our minds, we no longer relate to people as sexual conquests, nor do we judge people based on whether they are worthy of conquest. When we are no longer distracted by the thought of sex, we will be more present to whatever activity we are pursuing in the moment and will no longer have ulterior motives when we seek relationships with others. And when you do indeed engage in the sexual act, you will be more present to that activity as well. Your partner will be grateful for it.

The Spirit: Continence Serves Humanity

The highest form of sexual abstinence leads to the highest form of creativity: service to all of humanity and the Creative Spirit. When working in the realm of the spirit, abstinence from sex becomes not just a way to preserve energy and improve clarity of thought but a source of tremendous power. Mohandas Gandhi experimented with celibacy, and he led his entire country to independence. The potency of sexual essence is so great that it can move nations.

When we channel vitality wholly into productive works, we create an unrivaled opportunity to serve humanity. In no longer seeing others as possible sexual conquests, we embody a brotherly or sisterly love for all people. We seek people out not on the condition that they provide sexual gratification but to share the purity of our spirits.

Attaining control of this potent force gives the practitioner the feeling that they can accomplish anything; grounding this control in a spiritual practice like the One Plan will invariably lead to seeing each person as a pure and perfect spirit and wanting to serve that spirit. Anyone who questions the value of such a benefit might ask an elderly citizen of India what it was like living under British rule. Do you think someone from that time would find value in Gandhi's actions? If so, then perhaps there is something to this act of continence after all.

The Plan

As you explore continence, be sure to remember that everyone who has explored this practice—even Gandhi—has struggled with it. But also remember the significance of the rewards to be found.

The Realm of the Body

Addressing sexual continence at the most basic physical level is fairly straightforward. You will benefit from a physical practice of sexual abstinence if you release your sexual energy through orgasm on a regular basis and do so as often as you have the urge. Whether it's three times a week or three times a day, doing so less frequently will help your body retain health and vitality.

Your main task for this phase of your continence practice is to reduce your sexual release by half. If you have sex or masturbate six times a week, limit your activity to three times a week. If you release multiple times a day, limit your release to perhaps only once a day. You might not be quite so regular in your activity—some weeks you might feel more ardent than other weeks—so the general task is to reduce the release you have over the next two weeks. Then maintain that level of activity.

If you are in a committed relationship and feel that this reduced activity will be a source of tension between you and your partner, you can work to share the importance of this practice and how it will positively affect your life in other ways. It is important to pay more attention to your partner in moments previously devoted to sex, and to enjoy each other through other activities you have always intended to share but have put off.

Perhaps you are not in a relationship, but you invest considerable energy in seeking sexual release through encounters with others. You will benefit from a physical practice of continence if you invest time and effort into seeking sex without any interest in emotional connection. Additionally, you may be stimulating further release by seeking out sexual content, like pornographic films, or buying products because of the sexual way they were advertised. Spend these two weeks avoiding excursions centered on getting sex, a search for sexual content, and consumption of sexually advertised products—and continue to avoid doing so thereafter.

Because you will build up energy in response to this practice, another task for these two weeks is to find a physical activity that requires an investment of energy. This doesn't mean taking on just any sort of activity; find one you really connect with, which adds to your life and purpose. Below are some ideas to get you started:

- Discover nearby hiking trails, and devote time to hiking during the week.

- Take up a physical skill or discipline, like martial arts or horseback riding.

- Participate in organized physical activities, like taking dance classes or joining a gym.

- Complete a project you have put off for many years.

- Help your partner with a project.

- Renovate your home.

- Start an educational program you've always been interested in.

Pick the activity and explore it at least twice during these two weeks. When you partake in the activity, bring as much presence of mind to it as you can. Focus on each step as you hike, or on building the new project one task at a time. As you conduct your newfound physical activity, you will begin to relate to your body in a more aware and purposeful way that can also be applied to sexual activity. Make a commitment to participate in your new activity at least every couple of weeks as you progress on this new path.

The Realm of the Mind

As you develop your continence practice, you will find that you will have a greater investment in other activities as well as more platonic interest in people. These things happen in part because of your renewed energy and vitality, but they also come from a shift in your mind-set. If you start to direct your most creative energy into something other than release, you'll increasingly crave that higher form of satisfaction. If you start to see others not as conquests but as sources of spiritual connection, you'll share more tender and present moments.

You'll benefit from a mental practice of continence when you find that you experience half as much sexual gratification as you did in the last few years before beginning on this path. Likewise, if your sexual pursuits are no longer based entirely on release but are an expression of intimacy with another, you will find value in looking into the mental aspects of this practice.

Mental practice is very simple: For these two weeks, abstain from sex or sexual release. Instead use this time to invest greater energy into becoming better at some aspect of your life, be it your work, your family, creative expression, or some other activity of value. Just as you did when working in the realm of the body, you will store up energy as a result of abstinence. Pursuing other activities will not only enrich your life, but it will help you remain balanced in your thoughts.

There will be many moments when you may have thoughts like, "I really miss sex," "That person has a great body," or, in a less formal train of thought, "I really need to get laid." Use the Presence Practice each morning to ask yourself: What activity can I do with the restored energy I have from reduced sexual activity? Your newfound energy will create new opportunities that weren't conceivable when you began this journey. Spend five minutes considering how you could engage in your daily life with more focus and creativity. For example:

- Take up Ayurvedic cooking.

- Create an organic garden.

- Create with artistic media, such as paint, clay or ceramics, woodwork, or sculpture.

- Learn to build something, like furniture.

- Create new activities to do with your children.

- Find new ways that aren't sexual to express affection for your spouse.

- Volunteer, especially in a capacity that requires significant emotional investment (such as helping out at a hospital).

As you find new ideas through your Presence Practice for what to do with your preserved vitality, take steps to explore them. Commit yourself to taking at least one small step toward a new outlet for this energy before these two weeks are up.

The Realm of the Spirit

If you're struggling to see the value of withholding sexual release, then you will definitely benefit from exploring these ideas in the physical and mental realms. However, you'll know that you're going to benefit from exploring this practice within the spiritual realm if you find the prospect of exploring abstinence for a lengthy period of time—or for the rest of your life—to be filled with interesting possibilities. What might be possible with this sort of work?

Your practice at this level is to abstain from sex and sexual release for the next six to twenty-four months, putting all your energy into something that serves humanity and the Creative Spirit. This could mean turning your business into a not-for-profit endeavor and committing your work to the benefit of others. Or it could be supporting an organization that requires total immersion, like joining the Peace Corps. As you'll be storing up quite a bit of creative potency, you'll find that you need to serve more and more just to maintain balance. Large-scale endeavors will prove necessary for such an ambitious outlet. Regardless of the work that you do, you will assume greater community with the Creative Spirit. You will indeed become that spirit yourself.

Emerging as a Masterpiece

As you continue to build your practice, you may find that it's a challenge keeping up with all these different ideas. With time, though, you'll start to see that nonviolence, truthfulness, nonstealing, and the other components of this program aren't separate ideas at all. They're really just an assortment of tools for following the same basic path. With the practice of continence, you may experience frustration from time to time. But eventually you will see a rise in your energy and focus and be able to take on practices with greater follow-through and an ever-increasing sense of fulfillment.

Putting It Together

If you are practicing exclusively in the realm of the body, for these two weeks the tools will look like this:

- Determine how often you sexually release over the course of a typical two-week period, and reduce this to half.

- Avoid seeking out sexual encounters for the sake of gratification or seeking content of a sexual nature.

- Spend time at least twice during these two weeks participating in another physical activity that will lead to fulfillment and requires presence of mind.

And remember . . .

- Continue eating half as much processed food and unhealthy substances as you did prior to the program, and avoid eating during the last two hours of the day.

- Continue building your nonviolence, truthfulness, and nonstealing behaviors to the best of your ability.

If you are practicing exclusively in the realm of the mind, your daily practice over these two weeks will look like this:

- Avoid sexual release for these two weeks.

- Spend five minutes of your morning Presence Practice exploring possible outlets for your restored vitality. If something emerges as an ideal activity, take at least a first step toward this activity by the end of the two weeks.

And remember . . .

- Continue eating from the natural food groups, and avoid eating in the last five hours of the day and after 7 P.M.

- Continue your nonviolence, truthfulness, and nonstealing practices.

reversing the curse of the fearful

NONGREED

I MET MARIO THROUGH MY TV SHOW. MARIO RESPONDED TO THE PRODUCtion company when they put out a casting call to anyone in Los Angeles who was suffering from an ailment. Mario was hoping to get rid of a nasty case of psoriasis—red, leatherlike patches of excess skin all over his body. This condition lent itself well to television, for the visually alarming skin disorder definitely gave viewers something to respond to. Mario turned out to be the star of the pilot.

On the first day of filming, I showed up at Mario's home—a large house with lots of huge rooms. The furniture was beautifully coordinated, which led me to think that nothing in this palace existed by accident. As I got to know Mario, I learned that though he had worked in fashion design as a young man, he was now in information technology. He and his wife had two children in their pre- and early teens.

Ayurveda considers psoriasis to be an indication of accumulated toxins in the body. Since Mario's body was producing too much toxicity, the skin had to work extra hard to expel it, resulting in the leathery patches. The toxicity emerged in other ways as well, making him feel heavy and depressed as well as a little bit overweight. In treating Mario's condition, I prescribed the standard dietary changes, herbs, Yoga postures, and special treatments for the skin. I took him off coffee and alcohol. I even persuaded him to abstain from sex for a bit to help him redirect his vital energy to healing. He took very well to my program, he lost nine pounds after just a week of working together, and it brought a smile to his face.

One aspect of my work is to observe my client's living environment. Mario's immaculate house showed that he was a man of taste and refinement. But the grandeur of Mario's home was nothing compared to his wardrobe. He had dozens and dozens of shirts. He had drawers filled with pants. An entire wall of the closet was covered with sport coats and blazers, and when I asked him how many pairs of underwear he had, he said he owned a few hundred—a fact he knew off the top of his head.

"How long have you been collecting this stuff?" I asked him.

"Well, I actually don't collect it," he said. "If it sits in the closet for more than two years and I don't wear it, I probably won't wear it again. That's when I usually donate it."

We continued to talk as I looked over everything. I started to notice that the clothes varied in size.

"I used to be thinner," he said, "so things are different sizes."

"And now that you're losing weight again, you're not wearing the bigger clothes?"

"Right, now I won't need the larger sizes," he said.

I really liked Mario's impulse to donate the clothes he wasn't wearing, but his wardrobe wasn't getting any smaller, an indication of how many clothes he was buying.

"You have a deep attachment to your stuff," I said. He agreed.

I soon realized that Mario's current work in IT wasn't providing any outlet for the creativity he had used in the fashion industry. This enormous wardrobe was his compensation: instead of creating things, he bought other people's creations. Mario might have been consuming too much coffee and eating too many of the wrong foods, but this attachment to clothes was causing yet another form of toxicity. The accumulation of clothes was leading to accumulations in his skin. It also led to accumulations of negative energy in his mind, which accounted for the depression.

"What I'd like to do is have you donate some of your clothes to Operation New Hope," I said.

"What's that?"

"It's a local organization that helps at-risk youth finish their education and enter the workforce," I said. "Treatment comes in all forms, and you're holding on to a lot of material. Let's give that material away."

We brought out some large shopping bags and got to work. We put pants, shirts, jackets, and shoes into the bags. We stayed away from the underwear. Mario began to think like a stylist and picked out neutral clothes so the kids would have outfits appropriate for job interviews. He picked out a couple of very nice blue blazers, as well as some white shirts that would serve a variety of purposes. I was impressed that he focused on the styling and kept a light attitude about it, but then I realized something. Though he was putting plenty of clothes into the bags, they were all coming from certain parts of the closet.

"What about these over here?" I said, gesturing to a group of jackets at the end of the rack.

"Oh," he said. "Those are the smaller sizes. I'll actually be able to fit into those now that I'm losing weight again."

It became clear that Mario was putting only garments that no longer fit him into the bags, for he had no attachment to them. But if he didn't give away things he was attached to, he'd just be donating clothes he didn't want, as he had in the past.

"Here," I said, taking a lovely light wool coat off the rack next to me.

"This is a good one for the spring," he said, holding it in his hands. "This is nice."

Finally, he folded it up and put it in the bag. He continued to take more stuff off the rack, though the vibe had changed. Mario wasn't doing quite as well anymore.

We went to Operation New Hope. When we got there, we met the organization's director, Russell, as well as Zach, Juan, and Tito—three young men who were part of the program. Though they initially seemed shy because of the cameras filming for the show, the boys eventually described the steps they were taking toward careers, such as interning at a car dealership, learning to become a mechanic, and practicing to start a business. Mario began to ask them about the colors and patterns they preferred, giving them different things to try on.

He was in his element. He took out the blue blazers, the white shirts, and other garments. But these boys were barely out of their teens and yet to fully grow into their bodies, so it didn't surprise me when many of the clothes were too big. Mario had, after all, wanted to donate the clothing that fit him when he weighed more.

The light wool blazer and other smaller garments did fit, however. The boys still seemed shy in front of the cameras, but I could see a glimmer of satisfaction in Zach's eyes when he came out in a black pin-striped jacket, and Tito smiled as he modeled a pair of slacks. Juan just looked pleased with the whole thing. The biggest shift in energy, though, happened in Mario.

"I want to make sure you guys have what you need for your interviews," Mario said to them when they were all dressed up and looking slick. He then assured them that he would stay in touch with them as they took the next steps in searching for work.

"So, how are you doing?" I asked Mario on the car ride back to his house.

He started to shake his head. "I was having such a hard time putting some of those clothes in the bags. But not only did it feel incredible to see those guys wearing the outfits; it seems silly that I could have set them up with other ones if I hadn't wanted to hold on to the stuff that fit me. I wish I had brought them more."

Mario and I continued to work together for several more weeks, and as anyone watching the show's pilot could see, the journey we took together had results: he lost weight, he felt lighter and less depressed, and perhaps most notably, the patches on his skin were reduced by at least half. In some places, the psoriasis was completely gone.

The Pile of Berries

In the West we are taught to live like Mario. We collect trinkets. We stockpile food and supplies when they're on sale. Some of us are so prone to accumulating possessions that our homes are overrun by stuff—like the homes featured on *Hoarders*. We even collect relationships that hold little value in our day-to-day lives. Like Mario, we find that our bodies and lifestyles often suffer. Even though Mario donated some garments that he no longer wanted before working with me, he continued to accumulate even more. Why did Mario maintain such an enormous wardrobe? Like so many others, he lived in fear of not having what he needed. As a result, he accumulated what he didn't need at all.

Consider an animal living in the woods. Committed to survival, it forages for food to satisfy its hunger. A deer searches for fruits and leaves. A bird seeks out seeds and worms. A wolf hunts for deer and sheep. Once its hunger is satiated, the animal continues to live its life until it's hungry again. When a worm is sought out by a bird, it attempts to submerge itself into safety. When a deer is pursued by a wolf, it does what it can to escape the hunt. The cycle continues from there. At no point, though, does a deer store a pile of berries in case it's not able to find more the following day—nor does a wolf stick its latest kill in the fridge to pick at later when it wants a snack.

With the exception of animals like squirrels that store food for the winter or bears that eat extra food before they hibernate, hoarding food and possessions, and even having possessions at all, are distinctly human behaviors. To avoid daily trips to the supermarket, we store enough food for days at a time. To sustain our capacity to live and work, we need to own certain things. But many of us are so fearful of one day not finding berries—so to speak—that we hold on to as much as we can despite needing very little.

Aparigraha is the Yogic practice of nongreed, and it is the last of Patanjali's five abstentions. Our image of a greedy person is Ebenezer Scrooge counting his money without thinking about the welfare of others. Though miserly behavior is certainly one form of greed, the Yogic definition is any behavior through which people accumulate things they don't actually need. Stockpiling canned goods that won't be eaten for months is a form of greed. It is greedy to stick items in the garage to gather dust for years; what if someone else in the world could genuinely benefit from what you take for granted? Many people collect friends they don't trust and won't ever feel emotionally invested in because they fear being alone.

When we accumulate things we don't need, we have to invest energy in holding on to them. By owning many things, we create opportunities for loss ("What if someone took it?"). This only adds more fear, leading to a heavy, encumbering emotional burden. Life becomes about holding on to things—even toxins on the skin—instead of enjoying the moment.

Patanjali instructs us to avoid excessive behaviors in the body and mind and encourages us to use this simpler way of life to cultivate connection with the Creative Spirit. When we let go of our attachments to food, stuff, and people, we no longer hold on to those fears, we no longer burden others with our fears, and we welcome in a life of enrichment and abundance. When Mario unburdened himself of some of his wardrobe by giving it to the three boys, he felt lighter, experienced fulfillment, and wanted to give away even more.

A Different Type of Abundance

Practicing nongreed requires us to overcome fears of not having what we need in the future and to give away what we have hoarded from the past. When we overcome this fear, we welcome abundance into our lives through the physical, mental, and spiritual realms.

The Body: Nongreed Creates Lightness

As you can no doubt imagine, exploring nongreed within the realm of the body is the most straightforward aspect of this practice. To practice nongreed in the physical realm, we must let go of stockpiled food, inessential objects, and anything in our physical space that we don't use. When we let go of unnecessary objects, we also let go of the attachment and fear they inspire.

Now, this is not to say that we must own only things we need—like a single pot for cooking our dinner and a single plate to eat on. But we must let go of whatever we don't use—like a particularly valuable pair of earrings a woman may keep but never wears for fear of losing them. Holding on to things for no other reason than to not lose them just creates heaviness. When we live with only what we use in our day-to-day lives, we keep things simple. This creates lightness and affords us a far richer enjoyment of the world.

The Mind: Nongreed Creates Enrichment

Some people may live a generally spare existence, not owning too many things and not accumulating stuff. But not having a lot of stuff doesn't necessarily mean that there isn't any accumulation going on. A person could technically survive all alone, so they will be challenged by the mental realm of greed when they feel a significant attachment to situations and memories—be it holding on to objects of great sentimental value or even friendships that aren't fulfilling.

This becomes a mental experience because the fear is based less on losing one's relationship to one's surroundings ("I need objects to possess") than on fear of being in an undesirable situation ("What if I lose all connection to others and am left alone?").

When people we love pass away or leave us for good, we might covet mementos that remind us of them and make us feel as if we're still connected to them. Similarly, if we don't have fulfilling relationships, we may hang on to people we don't have a genuine connection to, don't particularly trust, or don't even like. But remaining attached to a memento or an uninspiring relationship only breeds more fear. If one were to lose the memento, would the person who left it no longer mean something to us? If we spend time by ourselves, does that mean we won't ever be in good company again? Perhaps it may help to look at this another way: if we spend our lives coveting objects that only remind us of loss or spend it in the company of those we don't like, aren't we blocking out more fulfilling situations that might come our way?

The Spirit: Nongreed Creates Peace

When material and situational attachments are gone, all that is left is community with the Creative Spirit. This is when we find joy in the simplest day, the simplest moment shared with another.

This is where we find peace.

The Plan

The program outlined for these two weeks of the One Plan is some of the most straightforward work but also some of the most challenging. In your commitment to this process, you will set the highest possible degree of happiness and fulfillment for yourself.

The Realm of the Body

Though many One Plan practices call on you to spend a set amount of time in an activity or permanently shift your behavior, the practice of nongreed in the realm of the body requires a finite amount of work with little follow-through beyond these two weeks. You know that you will benefit from this practice if you have a refrigerator filled with too much food, a pantry filled with cans and cartons you don't consume within a few weeks, and a house filled with stuff that hasn't been looked at or thought about for years. Your work is to let go of items you don't need and free up your living space. Over the course of these two weeks, you are going to clean house.

Getting rid of things can be not only emotional but time-consuming. Thus the work of these two weeks has been divided into areas so that no one purge is too daunting. Not only that, but each area, be it your refrigerator or your office, is divided into a two-day process. On the first day, take inventory of what you have, make decisions about what you plan to let go of, and gather together everything that makes the list. On the second day, physically remove the items from your home. Leftovers go into the trash, and old files are recycled. There are seven areas that are likely to need purging, and working on each for two days will fill up the two weeks of your focus on nongreed.

DAYS 1–2: THE REFRIGERATOR

When you look in most people's fridges, you'll find the door filled with half-empty jars, the shelves covered with leftovers, and more than one item past its expiration date. This image can serve as a metaphor for how people live in their own minds: cluttered, with far too many old things of no use. Clearing out your fridge will free you of items that you won't ever eat anyway. Will you ever actually use that last third of a bottle of barbeque sauce that you bought for a family cookout a year and a half ago? Foods like these were made so long ago that even if they were natural at one time, they no longer are. Spend Days 1–2 getting rid of whatever you don't think you're going to eat that week, and avoid accumulating items during these two weeks and beyond. Follow these steps:

- DAY 1: Go through your fridge and move everything that you know you're going to eat this week over to the side of the fridge opposite the door hinges. Take every jar, bottle, and plastic container with something old and inedible and move it to the opposite side or door.

- DAY 2: Take out everything that didn't make the cut, empty out the contents into the garbage or the disposal, and put the containers in the recycling bin to go out with the next pickup. If you have no recycling program, take the containers to the nearest processing center.

DAYS 3–4: THE PANTRY

The pantry is just a big refrigerator without the cold, in that it becomes a place for accumulating foods that won't be used in timely fashion. It's home to canned foods, boxes of mixes, and a variety of other prepackaged things. Not only have many of these foods been in their packages for a long time, but nearly all are unnatural and therefore not nourishing. Ideally, your pantry will only have simple, natural foods, such as nuts, seeds, grains (like rice and oats), dry legumes (like lentils), dry fruits, natural sweeteners, spices, and herbs. These are the only types of foods that don't lose their nutritional value right away, so they are the only ones to be kept. Spend Days 3–4 getting rid of anything in the pantry that isn't a natural food. Do this with the following steps:

- DAY 3: Create three categories for the items in your pantry: 1) half-consumed items that must be thrown out, 2) intact items, such as unopened canned goods, that can be donated to a food bank, and 3) natural foods that you plan to keep. Gather the category 1 items and place them in a large garbage bag; if the container is recyclable, empty the contents in the garbage and place the container in the recycling bin. Gather the category 2 items in boxes or shopping bags to be taken to a place that receives food donations.

- DAY 4: Take out the garbage as needed, and locate a place that receives food donations. Take the category 2 items to this location.

DAYS 5–6: THE BATHROOM

The bathroom is a place where we store many products that are not needed every day but are good to have around—like first-aid kits and cotton swabs. For many people, though, it is also a place where other things accumulate. This may include old bottles of mouthwash, dried-up makeup containers, and many other toiletry items that are no longer being used. These items should not be allowed to clutter up your bathroom. Spend Days 5–6 getting rid of them by taking the following steps:

- DAY 5: Take inventory of everything in the bathroom that you haven't used in six months, that has expired, or that is otherwise useless.

- DAY 6: Fill a garbage bag with the items you noted on Day 5, and take it out with the trash.

DAYS 7–8: THE OFFICE

Though it may be necessary to hold on to tax returns, mortgages, car leases, and other papers of contractual or legal significance, many of us also pack our office and desk spaces with many inessential items: old phone books, unusable scrap paper, puzzle books without any unused puzzles in them, dried-out rubber bands, and utility bills from the twentieth century. As none of these items have any further value, they've got to go. Spend Days 7–8 purging your office or desk space of anything that's been gathering dust for six months or more. Take the following steps:

- DAY 7: Create a pile of papers, phone books, memo pads, bills, files, and any other item that no longer has a practical or legal use. Shred documents that contain personal information if you would like to protect your privacy.

- DAY 8: Take everything out for recycling or to the trash if the discarded materials are not recyclable.

DAYS 9–10: CLOSETS AND DRESSERS

As these two weeks move along, it should become routine to purge your home of inessential items. This is why emptying out closets and dressers comes toward the end of these two weeks. We often feel very attached to clothes, just like Mario did, even if we haven't worn them in years. Though I'm by no means encouraging you to trade in your clothing for an orange swami robe, you will benefit from not being bogged down by garments you no longer use. There are many people who would be thrilled to own the clothes you have but don't wear anymore, so spend Days 9–10 letting go of them:

- DAY 9: Take everything that you haven't worn in the last three years off the rack and out of the drawers, including any clothes that no longer fit you. Odds are you won't wear them again. Place them in bags.

- DAY 10: Take the clothes to Goodwill, the Salvation Army, or some other place that takes donations. If you know of a place that would buy them from you and you would like to make some money, then you have the choice to pursue that instead. The most important thing, though, is to not spend too much time and energy trying to get as much as you can for them (as would happen if you spent a week preparing for a garage sale). The point here is to practice nongreed, and spending too much time trying to make money undermines the goal of lightening your load.

DAYS 11–12: THE GARAGE AND STORAGE

As you near the end of these two weeks of nongreed, you must face the heavy lifting: clearing out your garage or extra storage. Though some tools, appliances, and other items are likely necessary for your day-to-day life, there are also many things—like dried-up makeup and old utility bills—that no longer serve a purpose. This can include anything from a box of old toys your children outgrew ten years ago to an extra bucket of spackle that your contractor didn't use for a renovation at about the same time your child outgrew the toys. This step of your living space purge is one of the more ambitious ones, as it will likely require you to make some tough decisions about what you do and do not need—but it also may require some actual heavy lifting. For Days 11–12, take the following steps:

- DAY 11: Go through your garage and storage space and write down everything that you plan to get rid of, separating items into two columns: column A for things you are throwing away, and column B for things you're giving away. Try to keep the number of things that go in Column A to a minimum, as it will ultimately become landfill. Anything that can be recycled should be processed accordingly. For everything in Column B, write down where you plan to donate the item.

- DAY 12: Load up your car with everything you plan to throw away or recycle, and take it to the dump. If you have too much for your vehicle or you don't have a vehicle, order a large trash receptacle and fill it up at your home before having it taken away. Deliver whatever you're giving away, and make arrangements for those who are picking up items to come by within the next week.

- SPECIAL NOTE: Given the size and ambition of this process, it is likely that getting everything accomplished will take more than two days. Even if it takes you longer to get everything done, be sure to give yourself a deadline so it is taken care of within two weeks of Day 12. Otherwise, it will hang over your head and become a burden.

Days 13 and 14 are focused on purging your library or bookshelves. If the progression of these two weeks of nongreed is that the items are harder and harder to let go of (throwing out a half-empty jar of pickles is easier than throwing out, say, an old piano), then why does the library come last? Given that you're reading this, you clearly assign at least some value to books. You may even find books to be one of the most valuable things in existence. However, how many books do you own that you haven't picked up and read for years? How many books do you own that you haven't even read at all? Though bookcases filled with books may seem pretty and scholastic looking, they are another form of material excess that is likely bogging you down. Though having books to read can be incredibly valuable, having books that aren't read is not. Spend Days 13–14 purging your shelves of books you no longer read, using the following steps:

- DAY 13: Make a stack of all the books, magazines, or newspapers you haven't read in the last five years and don't have any plans of reading in the next year. If a book has particular sentimental value (such as a book inscribed to you by a loved one), then letting go of it is more of a mental practice. Otherwise, a book can likely be replaced down the line if you really need to read it again.

- DAY 14: Take the books to a place that accepts donations or to a used bookstore that will buy them from you.

By the end of these two weeks, you will likely own considerably fewer things. If someone opens your fridge, you will probably receive questioning looks about its barren appearance. No matter what happens, though, be sure to sustain this minimal level of material ownership so as to keep the lightness created by an ongoing practice of nongreed. If, a year from now, your home looks like it did at the beginning of Week 9, you'll benefit from going through the purge once again.

The Realm of the Mind

Whereas the physical practice of nongreed was a rigorously structured process, the mental practice is anything but. You will benefit from a mental practice if you own and keep only items that you have specific use for. If you are in this position, you will likely benefit from overcoming fears based on situations more than material survival. In the first week of your nongreed practice, find an object that you have particular sentimental attachment to. It may remind you of someone or inspire memories of an experience you particularly enjoyed. If the object could be of value to someone else, like a piece of inherited antique jewelry, give it away or sell it and donate the funds to a cause close to your heart. If it is only of value to you, like an old photo you keep of someone who has passed away, have a ritual or a personal ceremony that allows you to let it go (by burning it, burying it, etc.). The object may be gone, but your memories of that person are not. Use this practice as a way to let go of unhealthy attachments, while still enjoying how that person enriched your life.

For the second week of your practice, use the Presence Practice each day to consider a person who is currently in your life with whom you have a troubled relationship. This may be a relative with whom you have an ongoing tension, a friend you tolerate but don't particularly enjoy, or even someone you've known for a long time but only spend time with out of a sense of obligation. When we maintain such a relationship, we do so because we fear being alone or being thought unkind. This fear adds to our burden. Spend your five minutes of Presence Practice asking yourself the following questions:

- How might my struggles and this other person's struggles be similar?

- How might our struggles be different?

- What might this person be here to teach me or to remind me of?

Then, on the seventh day, make a decision to either reach out and have a conversation with this person or sever ties and move on. If you choose to create a more significant connection, you will now have another person in your life with whom you share a meaningful bond. If you choose to let that person go, you will make room for more relationships that inspire you to live a more fulfilling life. Either way, however, you must remove yourself from relationships and situations that don't serve you.

The Realm of the Spirit

You're probably familiar with the images of Tibetan monks who wear nothing but simple red robes, Indian swamis who wear nothing but orange robes, or even Gandhi, who wore a simple ensemble of homespun cloth. Each of these people let go of material possessions for the sake of fostering a relationship with humanity and the Spirit. You will benefit from practicing nongreed in the realm of the spirit if you are ready to let go of all your clothing, except one outfit, as well as all other possessions, sustaining yourself on the barest of essentials.

To practice nongreed in this realm, spend these two weeks giving away whatever you don't need to sustain your day-to-day life. If you own a home, welcome others in to stay with you, and allow them to use the home as their own. Or donate land you own to a nonprofit organization or start your own. In this realm, all things are owned by everybody and nobody. Rather than collecting possessions, begin to gather and build community. Here, owning nothing, you really will have chipped away all of the unnecessary marble to leave only the essential stone, allowing the perfection of your own personal masterpiece to shine its light onto the world.

Emerging as a Masterpiece

As the last of the abstentions, your practice of nongreed will cap off a significant aspect of grounding your practice. By the end of these two weeks, you will be living in a clutter-free home, experiencing far greater lightness than you did before you began Week 1, and if you have begun exploring the realm of the mind, you will be letting go of emotionally significant things as well. This simpler, lighter situation you've created for yourself will allow you to be more open to the five observations that follow over the next ten weeks of the program.

Putting It Together

If you are practicing exclusively in the realm of the body, for the first two weeks that you practice nongreed your routine will look like this:

- Spend these two weeks removing inessential items from the seven areas of your home.

And remember . . .

- Continue eating half as much processed food and unhealthy

substances as you did earlier, avoid eating during the last two hours of the day, and release your sexual essence half as often as before.

- Continue building your nonviolence, truthfulness, and nonstealing behaviors to the best of your ability. Replace seeking out sex with another physical activity that requires presence of mind.

If you are practicing exclusively in the realm of the mind, your daily practice over these two weeks will look like this:

- Spend the first week finding something of sentimental value to let go of.

- Spend the second week using the Presence Practice to decide whether to build or let go of a troublesome relationship.

And remember . . .

- Continue eating natural foods, refrain from eating in the last five hours of the day and after 7 P.M., and continue limiting your sexual behavior.

- Continue your nonviolence, truthfulness, and nonstealing practices, and avoid sexual thoughts as well.

returning to perfection

PURITY

MY FIRST STEP TOWARD BECOMING AN AYURVEDA AND YOGA therapist was to participate in a Yoga teacher training with the Integral Yoga Institute in New York City. The training lasted six months, and though much of the course was focused on teaching us how to instruct students in the physical postures, there were other aspects of the course as well.

Integral Yoga was created by Sri Swami Satchidananda. Satchidananda came to the United States in the 1960s and founded Yogaville, an ashram in Virginia. Toward the end of my training, the institute shuttled the trainees down to Yogaville to highlight additional aspects of the Yogic path. During this time, we learned about practices beyond postures and got an opportunity to be outside in nature—something New Yorkers rarely do.

My fellow trainees and I were an interesting array of urban cowboys looking to create new experiences for ourselves. One lovely girl seemed to belong in a crystal shop where she could burn incense sticks all day. One dude was a musician who, though rather chill on the outside, seemed to be up for anything. A young woman who was born in Brooklyn—and mentioned her background often—looked at any situation in which there was another person around as an opportunity to chat. As is probably easy to imagine, the bus ride to Virginia was interesting.

The Satchidananda Ashram in Yogaville consisted of several buildings that formed a lotus flower, with the center's temple in the middle of the flower. During the week, we learned about breathing practices, performed devotional practices like mantra, studied the Yoga Sutras, and helped clean the temple in an act of selfless service known as *seva*. Each morning, we woke up at five o'clock. and participated in a variety of rituals and routines that gave us further insight into the Yogic path.

About halfway through the week, we were to participate in something known as a *kriya*. These techniques, which are a part of Yoga philosophy, are cleansings done by ingesting various substances or simply using the breath in a cleansing way. The specific *kriya* we were going to do was for cleansing the stomach, the lungs, the head region, and the body as a whole. To do this, we would induce vomiting.

We learned a technique that involved drinking warm salt water until our stomachs were completely filled. Taking in any further salt water would cause us to vomit. The salt water would bring up bile and mucus, and the gastrointestinal tract would undergo detoxification. They told us that we would feel lighter and deeply cleansed as a result of this technique.

To represent the purification that was about to happen, our teachers had us dress all in white. They had us come outside to the gardens to practice on the pathway among the flowers and bushes. I was there to learn, so I began to drink as soon as they presented us with the water. Some of my fellow trainees, not so much.

"I don't really know about this," said the usually chill musician.

"It would be a shame to get vomit all over these lovely white clothes," said the girl who belonged in the crystal shop.

"You want us to do WHAT?" said the girl from Brooklyn.

Eventually, though, they came around and started to drink as well. At first I did fine, downing cup after cup. But then, after about four cups, I started to slow down.

"If this was like knocking back shots, I'd be on my sixteenth," said the musician after three cups.

"I can't do this," said crystal girl after four.

"This is horrible," said the girl from Brooklyn after five. "At first it tasted like wonton soup but now it's just—"

I looked up from my cup at the girl.

"Now it's just—" she said again.

Then she ran over to the bushes.

"WHOOO-AACHK."

The crystal lady was next.

"BLLLEEECAACK."

The musician found a nice marsh marigold bush to offer his fertilizer to.

"HHOONNKE."

More and more of my fellow trainees started spewing up their salt water, while the girl from Brooklyn just kept chatting away. I had no idea that somebody could talk and vomit at the same time. By this time, I was suffering through my fifth cup. I knew my stomach wasn't completely full, but my mind wasn't cooperating and letting me see it through to the end. Rather than allow it to happen with a full stomach, I found a bush of my own, pressed my fingers to the back of my tongue, and regurgitated my morning's activities onto the ground. The bile that came up fit in nicely with the plant's surrounding soil.

"The last time that happened," said the musician with a laugh, "I had had three Long Island Ice Teas. Dude, let's do that again."

Maybe he really was up for anything after all. But at least that morning, I was not. Maybe next time.

Greater Health and Vitality

Looking back at my experience in Yogaville, it's no coincidence that I went through the *kriya* practice among people who made references to Long Island Ice Tea and knocking back shots. Here in the West, we seek out every gratification we can find in the pursuit of pleasure and entertainment. You likely have spent more than one evening of your life stimulating every one of your senses by eating lots of food, taking a few choice narcotics, and of course, knocking back some shots. After a night of indulgence, you've probably woken up the next morning (afternoon?) with headaches, gas, and a wish that you had made different choices the night before. After having sought out every kind of physical gratification, you then spend the rest of the day feeling miserable and just trying to recover.

This misery in the body leads to misery in the mind. Perhaps after your night of drinking you are nursing a hangover and get mad at a friend for talking too loudly—even though they're talking at the same volume they usually do. You say something about how annoying they are, they get offended, and then suddenly you're having a fight about how you drink too much and how your friend is too judgmental and controlling. Had you avoided the night of indulgence, you would never have felt off balance and you never would have gotten mad at your friend or anyone else for their volume.

Though it's kind of funny to think about Long Island Ice Tea in the context of a solemn practice done in white clothing, it also paints a significant picture: In Western cultures, we are destroying our bodies and minds through the many harmful ways our culture has promoted to gratify our cravings. Furthermore, we take in all sorts of impurities through polluted air, polluted sounds, and the chemicals that invariably find their way into the food we eat—even if we buy organic foods at the grocery store. And yet, how many of us make time to take care of our bodies in any meaningful way? How many of us shortchange our diets by stopping off for a quick bite at a fast food restaurant instead of taking twenty minutes to prepare fresh food? How many of us are willing to invest even a little time reversing the harmful stimuli that are thrown at us every day? With these harmful experiences, our bodies and minds grow weaker and are more susceptible to illness and suffering. The more we experience suffering, the further we are from experiencing happiness and peace.

Over the first ten weeks of the One Plan, you have likely picked up on the nature of Patanjali's concepts through the realm of the spirit. Each practice within this realm reflects the belief that each of us has a perfect spirit. When this spirit becomes fully realized, it allows us to shed light and love onto the world. To live in reflection of this aspect of ourselves is to live in perfection. Purity, known by the Sanskrit word *saucha,* is the act of cleansing body and mind so that they may provide a more balanced container or temple for the spirit. Rather than allowing our bodies and minds to grow weaker, we find greater health and vitality through the act of purification. As the first of Patanjali's five observations and the next aspect of this path, it allows the natural purity of the spirit to shine throughout our lives.

Though the story about the vomiting down at Yogaville was about an act of body purification, there was clearly a lot of mind stuff we had to get rid of to be open to such an experience. As you will soon see, the distinction between purifying the body and purifying the mind can often be difficult to make.

The Other Side of Nonviolence

As an abstention, nonviolence is defined by avoiding harmful behaviors. In contrast, purification is defined by embracing beneficial ones. Experiencing purity within the realms of the body, the mind, and the spirit is not about what we won't do, but about what we will.

The Body: Purification for Cleansing

When we pursue a physical nonviolence practice, we abstain from behaviors that harm the body, such as eating poorly, drinking alcohol, and smoking cigarettes. Our physical purification process is based on participating in methods and modalities that strengthen the body's capacity for detoxification and cleanliness. This can happen through any number of cleansing methods. Much like the cleansing my fellow teacher trainees and I did that day in Yogaville, it can include taking herbs that purge and strengthen the body, or simply sipping hot water in the morning to help flush out impurities from the night before. Modern approaches teach us that detoxification means completing a strong bodily cleanse defined by extreme measures. But Ayurvedic and Yogic principles of cleansing the body are different. The ancient systems state that our bodies will always have toxins in them—even after a cleanse—so it's best to do them in a softer way but more frequently. These systems teach us that once we clean the body and mind, we must nourish them back to a state of strength.

In this section of the Yoga Sutras, Patanjali explains that through purification, we become disinterested in our bodies. When the body is clean, he says, we have less interest in seeking out ways to dirty it once again. We protect the body from contamination, which is like abstaining from physical violence toward ourselves. But why look at purification of the body in this way? If we dirtied our bodies, surely we could go out and detoxify them again? Wouldn't that cancel out anything that makes the body impure?

As an observation rather than an abstention, purification relies on our interest in preparing the body for the higher practices along the Yogic path. To have a pure body is to have not simply a detoxified body but one that is readily available to sit and conduct practices like concentration and meditation. This practice of purity helps us become proactive in taking care of the body. With a conscious and deliberate effort to remain pure in the body, there will be far more energy for the more ambitious practice of finding purity in the mind.

The Mind: Purification for Fostering Clarity

As we purify the body, we start to crave purer thoughts. When we consider the path we've followed so far, each practice underlines the idea that our minds can undermine our happiness. We exhibit harmful thoughts, such as those in the example of one friend being mad at the other after waking up with a hangover. When we have these harmful thoughts, we're filling ourselves with destructive feelings that then undermine our well-being as a whole. This further distracts us from the ultimate purity that is our spirit. When we abstain from harmful thoughts, we allow ourselves to live in peace and are inspired to share that peace with others. The act of purifying the mind helps us retain that peaceful place and allows the mind to be more resilient when adversity strikes.

How do we do this? Just as we drink hot water or take herbs to flush out the body, we use certain methods to purify our minds. One of these methods is mantra. Mantra is a phrase or a lengthier passage of text that, in the Yogic tradition, is based on the Sanskrit language. The sounds and thoughts created by reciting certain Sanskrit words cause vibrations that have a purifying resonance in the mind. The purity of these words cleanses the mind of its toxic thoughts, much like drinking water purifies the body's channels of their toxicity. This leads to a less preoccupied mind, and as we commit more and more of our lives to experiencing such a state, we commit more and more of our lives to purity.

The Spirit: The Source of Purity

With pure bodies and minds, we pave the way to fully realizing our spirit. A spirit cannot be purified, for it is already pure. It is already perfect. The body is no longer burdened by the harmful stimuli we encounter during our day-to-day life, and the mind is no longer burdened by the angry or conflicted thoughts we previously had toward ourselves and others. When we embody purity, we are ready to share and connect with the rest of the world that part of us which is already perfect. Neither harsh words nor destructive actions from a person who is suffering can hurt us. Nothing can hurt our spirit, for no matter how broken our bodies or how distorted our minds, our spirit will be pure now and forever. This is what living in purity truly is.

The Plan

Can you imagine what would happen if you tried to design a bridge across a river without learning a single thing about engineering? The bridge, if it could even be built, would collapse before the first car could cross it. Similarly, the traditions of Yoga and Ayurveda have methods for purifying body and mind, but without proper training under the guidance of an experienced teacher, they can be misused and perhaps lead to the Yogic equivalent of a collapsed bridge. The techniques below will help you purify your body and mind, but they are ultimately only introductory practices. However, it's a start.

The Realm of the Body

The following techniques will help you purify your body and strengthen selected organs. You will benefit from pursuing the realm of the body if you don't already make daily use of these techniques.

The following techniques are the first component you'll add to your morning routine. For this practice, you will need water, salt, neem or tulsi powder, other herbs as listed below, sesame oil (or almond or olive oil), castor oil, ghee, a toothbrush, a tongue scraper, small bowls, and a small bottle with an eyedropper top.

WEEKS 11–12: Each day, drink hot water first thing in the morning. This will serve as a replacement for coffee, tea, or other stimulants, helping to cleanse the body and strengthen the digestion.

As you drink your hot water, use the Presence Practice to work on not suppressing natural urges, including yawns, sneezes, burps, and flatulence. These are natural responses to what is happening in the body, including by-products that have built up during the night. Suppressing them keeps in toxins that are trying to leave the body. Many diseases start this way, because pushing back whatever is causing these urges alters the flow of air and intoxicates the system. When you pursue your five minutes of Presence Practice, simply ask yourself if you suppress any of these urges, and which situations inspire such behavior.

Then, whenever you feel an urge coming along, be sure to let it happen even if you have to run away and be on your own for a moment.

Over these two weeks, you are to gradually work toward a morning ritual of cleaning and nourishing the orifices of your body, such as your mouth and your eyes. Cleaning the orifices purges the body of dirt and toxicity, and oiling them helps strengthen the associated bones and muscles. Once you've worked your way through several cleaning and oiling techniques, you will move on to a light purgation and the use of herb teas. I introduce these methods gradually over the two weeks, giving you every other day to ground yourself in the new technique before presenting another. Be sure, however, to add each routine to the previous one, unless otherwise noted. I have broken down each task by the day(s) they are introduced, providing instruction accordingly.

DAYS 1–2: INTRODUCE CLEANING AND OILING THE MOUTH

The dental products we use in modern Western culture are filled with chemicals and additives that may have disinfecting properties but don't strengthen the gums or teeth. The following routine helps free the teeth of food particles and any harmful bacteria living in the mouth while nourishing the gums and teeth.

- Gargle with salt water to clean and disinfect the mouth. You can also do this with a quarter cup of sesame oil, which will help remove mucus and keep the throat strong and ulcer-free.

- Mix one teaspoon of sesame oil and a quarter teaspoon of neem or tulsi powder in a small bowl. You can replace the neem or tulsi with one drop of the essential oil of clove, sage, or oregano if you like. You can make a larger batch of this mixture all at once to be used daily over time.

- Use a conventional soft toothbrush or your fingers to brush the mixture into the teeth, much like you do with modern toothpaste.

- After brushing, take a tongue scraper and scrape the tongue with a stroke starting at the back of the tongue and ending at the front. Repeat this stroke four or five times.

DAYS 3–4: INTRODUCE CLEANING AND OILING THE NOSE

We often get dirt and excess mucus in the nose from pollution in the air or an unhealthy diet. The following routine cleans the nose and lubricates it so it doesn't dry out. This reduces the amount of dirt that finds its way into the nasal passages.

- Mix warm water with a pinch or two of rock, sea, or regular salt in a small bowl until the salt is dissolved.

- Cup the hand and pour a small amount of water into the cupped hand.

- Cover one nostril, sniff the salt water up the open nostril, and blow it out.

- Repeat with the other nostril.

- Dip your pinky finger into a little bit of ghee or sesame, olive, or almond oil, and massage the oil into the inside of each nostril.

DAYS 5–6: INTRODUCE OILING THE EYES

Our eyes can grow weak and tired, particularly given how much time we spend staring at electronic screens. Ghee, known also in the West as clarified butter, has a nourishing and strengthening effect. The following routine strengthens the eyes. *Note that this is only practiced once a week.*

- Melt a small amount of ghee, allowing it to cool until it's no longer hot but is still liquid.

- Take three or four drops of ghee on a spoon, tilt the head back, place the spoon just above the corner of the eye, and let one or two drops of ghee fall into the eye.

- Repeat with the other eye.

- Rotate the eyes around in each direction for a few seconds.

- Dab the eyes with tissue to remove the excess ghee.

DAY 7: SPEND DAY 7 REINFORCING THE FIRST TWO ROUTINES

DAY 8: INTRODUCE OILING THE EAR

There are a number of fragile, tiny bones inside the ear that will benefit from the strengthening properties of oil. The following routine will ensure that your ears function properly and remain healthy throughout your life. *Note that it is only necessary to practice this part of the routine once a month.*

- Take some sesame oil and put it in a small jar with an eyedropper top.

- Retain about five drops of oil in the dropper, tilt your head to one side, and squeeze the drops into your ear. Remain like this for three to five minutes.

- Tip your head in the opposite direction while holding a tissue to the ear so as to catch the excess oil.

- Repeat with the other ear.

DAY 9: INTRODUCE OILING THE ANUS

With the strain and rubbing created by moving one's bowels and the wiping that follows, the anus can develop hemorrhoids and other problems of dryness in later life. The following routine will help you avoid such ailments. *Note that this is only practiced once a week.*

- Pour about a half teaspoon of sesame oil in your right hand. Dip a finger from your left hand into the oil.

- Rub the oil onto the outside of the anus first. Then dip the finger into the oil again, enter about an inch into the anus with the finger, and rub the oil inside. Repeat until all the oil in the hand has been used. Be gentle and slow, as the membrane is quite fragile.

DAY 10: SPEND DAY 10 REINFORCING THE FIRST TWO ROUTINES

DAY 11 (END OF DAY 10): TAKE CASTOR OIL OR TRIPHALA

Castor oil and triphala are highly effective but natural ways to clean the colon. The amount you take is based on your body size and needs. Here I have suggested a small amount that everyone will benefit from, but you can use more or less depending on your daily needs and your body's reaction to the herbs.

- The night before Day 11, take one half to one tablespoon of castor oil or one to three teaspoons of triphala two hours before going to bed. Follow the castor oil with half a cup of warm water. Mix the triphala with one cup of warm water.

- If effective, you should feel the need to move your bowels first thing the next morning. Depending on your body's sensitivity, the castor oil may act much faster.

- Again, this can be a powerful therapy depending on the amount of herb you take, *so be sure to practice this routine no more than once or twice a week.*

- If you have significant, long-term issues with constipation, consult a trained Ayurvedic practitioner to resolve this issue in a guided way.

- If you are a woman, avoid doing this during your monthly cycle or while pregnant.

DAYS 12–14: TAKE PURIFYING HERBS

The Ayurvedic system of medicine has cataloged hundreds upon hundreds of plants that have medicinal properties in their leaves, roots, fruits, and other components. The use of these plants forms the basis of Ayurvedic herbology, which is used to treat all sorts of ailments and imbalances.

Herbs that have a balancing, strengthening, and purifying effect on the body include tulsi, ginger, turmeric, haritaki, licorice, ashwaghanda, shatevari, coriander, cumin, black pepper, fennel, cardamom, and amalaki. For Days 12 to 14 of this practice, you are to take two or three of these herbs prepared as a tea using the following steps:

- Place a half teaspoon of two or three herbs in a coffee mug. If you prefer to put the herbs in a tea bag, that is fine.

- Boil water on the stove (never the microwave!), and pour it into the mug. Let the tea steep for at least seven minutes before drinking.

- Complete this routine once in the late morning, perhaps after breakfast, and at least once later in the day.

Once you have completed this two-week introduction to morning purification practices, continue this routine each morning on an ongoing basis. Remember to oil the eyes only once a week, to oil the anus only once a week, to ingest castor oil only once or twice a week, and to oil the ears only once a month.

The Realm of the Mind

Mantra is a path to purification of the mind. You will benefit from exploring this realm after you've sustained a daily purity ritual for at least six months or a year.

WEEK 11: *Practice the Gayatri Mantra.* You have likely heard of mantra as a method for training the mind. The practitioner repeats Sanskrit words to fill the mind with spiritually beneficial sound vibrations. Sanskrit syllables have a therapeutic quality whether they're spoken aloud or said internally. One of the most common mantras is "om," which is traditionally considered to represent all of creation. You will begin the mental practice of purification by practicing a very powerful mantra known as the Gayatri Mantra. This mantra is known for its cleansing effect on the mind.

The Gayatri Mantra must be pursued with great reverence and devotion. The text of this mantra is:

Om bhur bhuvah svahah
tat savitur varenyam
bhargo devasaya dhimahi
dhiyo yo naha pracodayat

The mantra provides the practitioner with an opportunity to connect with the Spirit and stay on the path of realizing a divine light. You may chant the mantra out loud using online aids or guided meditation recordings, or it can be internalized and said to yourself. You are to practice Gayatri Mantra each morning after conducting your purification ritual for the body. For Week 11, take the following steps to incorporate the recitation of the Gayatri Mantra into your daily practice:

DAYS 1–2: Use whatever technique works best for you to memorize the text of the mantra. This may be writing out each line on an index card and repeating the words to yourself again and again, then testing your memory of the words before flipping the card over and reading it, or some other technique. Spend at least ten or fifteen minutes each of these two days learning the mantra.

DAYS 3–7: Incrementally increase the time you either say the mantra out loud or repeat it to yourself. On Day 3, start with six minutes, adding a minute each day until you're practicing for ten minutes on Day 7. Continue this practice each day thereafter. Be sure to sit on the floor in a cross-legged position or, if this is too difficult, sit on the edge of a chair. Keep your spine erect.

WEEK 12: *Avoid touching people for a week.* The sutra that discusses this practice mentions that purity creates a disinterest in our own and other people's bodies. When we seek the path of purity that ultimately leads to self-realization, the human body becomes simply a vessel for attaining that state. To explore this idea, spend this week avoiding physical contact with other people. This means handshakes and other physical greetings in addition to more intimate exchanges, such as hugs, kisses, and sexual activity. Rather than shaking hands, offer the traditional Indian greeting of *namaste*—which means "My divine light acknowledges the divine light in you"—with your hands in prayer position. If you feel self-conscious about this socially unconventional practice, take a moment to explain what you are doing. Spend this week reflecting on the significance of your body in your life, and to what extent you feel attachment to its role in your time here on earth. The practice is not to avoid people but to communicate with others through the mind. This experience will help you become aware of how we constantly use the body to connect on a physical level. At the end of the week, resume normal physical contact, at which point your deeper attachments will come to light.

The Realm of the Spirit

Exploring the realm of the spirit through a purity practice is almost redundant, as those who exist in or are well on their way into this realm need not concern themselves with purity—their community with their spirit is purity itself. However, moving from the realm of the mind into the realm of the spirit will be assisted by lifestyle adjustments. Your devotion to this path will benefit from the guidance of a guru who is in a position to give you the best mantra and other practices to use for spiritual growth. Living this way in Western culture requires a lot of discipline, so you will benefit from moving to a more secluded environment. Your work may reflect what follows, or it may take a different shape. You will benefit from exploring this realm if these lifestyle changes suit your nature and come naturally, otherwise you will suffer unnecessarily.

In a significant physical cleanse, the stomach is purged of excess bile and mucus. One way to do this is to consume several cups of warm salt water (known as *Kunjal Kriya*) to fill the stomach and induce vomiting. The intensity of this practice dictates that it should be done no more than once a month without supervision. This *kriya* can be practiced by taking the following steps:

- Practice first thing in the morning, after going to the bathroom but before any other routine.

- On the stove, prepare a small saucepan with about half a gallon of water and about two teaspoons salt.

- Warm the water without letting it get too hot to drink.

- Drink the salt water until the stomach is full. This may be eight cups or more.

- When it is impossible to drink any more, vomit the water into the toilet, either by natural urge or by using your fingers to instigate a gag reflex.

- When bile comes up, you are done.

To further your practice, avoid touching anyone for months or years. This is so all of the different practices that have been accumulated in the body are not lost through touch. This, like any practice sustained over lengthy periods, will liberate you from physical and mental bondage.

Regardless of how your time on earth takes shape, your practice of purity within the realm of the spirit will be a constant reminder to yourself and others that our souls are not only pure but eternally the joyful product of the divine force responsible for all life.

Emerging as a Masterpiece

Shifting from the abstentions to the observations means that, instead of removing behaviors, you'll be spending more time practicing actions that will then be sustained over time. You will also begin to experience immediate changes, such as the rejuvenating benefits of the morning purity routine. Take note of how you're feeling when you clean and oil your orifices. Does your mouth feel cleaner? Does your nose seem less dry? You will see greater and greater benefit from these practices as you become accustomed to this part of your daily ritual.

Putting It Together

If you are pursuing this program entirely in the realm of the body, for these two weeks your routine will be as follows:

- Begin to incorporate the purity practices into your morning routine, including drinking hot water. Here is a suggested schedule:

  - Go to the bathroom.

  - Drink hot water (and for these two weeks, use the Presence Practice to avoid repressing natural urges, such as yawning and burping).

  - Clean the orifices (mouth, eyes, etc.).

- Remember to limit certain techniques to a weekly or monthly basis as noted.

- Take herbal tea twice a day to build strength and cleanliness.

And remember . . .

- Continue eating half as much processed food and unhealthy substances as you did before, avoid eating during the last two hours of the day, and release your sexual essence half as often as you did before Week 7. Continue to avoid accumulating possessions.

- Continue building your nonviolence, truthfulness, and nonstealing behaviors to the best of your ability. Continue participating in a physical activity that requires presence of mind at least once every two weeks.

If you are practicing exclusively in the realm of the mind, your daily practice over these two weeks will look like this:

- Practice the Gayatri Mantra. Conduct this practice after completing the orifice-cleaning ritual.

- For the second of these two weeks, avoid physical contact with others.

And remember . . .

- Continue eating natural foods, avoid eating in the last five hours of the day and after 7 P.M., and continue to have sex in moderation.

- Continue your nonviolence, truthfulness, and nonstealing practices, and avoid sexual thoughts. Continue to let go of your attachments to people and situations that you are keeping out of fear.

the great secret

CONTENTMENT

BACK IN MY FASHION DAYS, I KNEW A PHOTOGRAPHER WHO REALLY wanted a family. She had tremendous talent and expressed herself beautifully in her work. Even as early as her twenties, she was able to capture a simple expression in a way that inspired the viewer to experience the photo not just as an image but as a story. If you were to look at her life through her career, you would think she had it all. But though she often went out on dates, she rarely met anyone she felt even remotely interested in. Even though she really wanted to settle down and have a husband and kids, she couldn't bring herself to compromise on what she wanted. I respected her unwillingness to give up on her ideals.

Before I left the industry, we fell out of touch. I remained in New York, and she went to work on the West Coast. I didn't run into her again until years later, when we were both in our midthirties. I was still in New York and was finding my way through the beginning of the Yogic path. She was still working as a photographer but had shifted into less fashion-driven work and was focusing instead on high-end merchandising. She was also still single. She was living in San Francisco and had had a series of relationships, but nothing had inspired her to start a family. I noted that she didn't look disappointed when she said this, but she did seem somewhat tired.

"One thing I've realized," she said, "is that I need to stop being so limited in how I see things."

"Oh?" I said. The practices I had begun pursuing on the Yogic path were steering me toward a more detached mind-set. I didn't want to be limited in how I saw things, either.

"Yeah," she said. "I've come to realize that I can't really limit my search for a husband to just where I'm living. I recently decided that I need to move to whatever city will allow me to be with someone."

"Oh," I said again. She wasn't talking about the same kinds of limitations as I encountered on the Yogic path. After she said this, I noted that what I thought was her seeming tired was more likely her feeling resigned. Her inability to meet her soul mate meant she would have to marry a less-than-ideal spouse if she was going to start a family.

Soon after, I went to India and lost touch with many people I knew in the States, including her. But I didn't let go of that image of her resignation. I know if she had been a photographer of her own life in that moment she would have been able to capture an image that told a story. It would have been an image of a woman who was setting herself up for a life filled with one simple but difficult feeling: discontentment.

Revealing the Secret

Have you ever gone through something like my photographer friend's experience? If you've ever felt that your life would be totally manageable if you just made $10,000 more a year, or fallen in love with a new piece of clothing that you felt you absolutely had to have, or felt that what you had at that moment wasn't quite enough to make you happy, then the answer is yes. My friend enjoyed a successful and creative career that she had a natural talent for, found new ways to explore life in different cities and in different professional capacities, and likely had many more opportunities to explore. And yet, when I saw her in New York, she didn't seem happy with much of anything. She seemed disappointed, and the value of her life seemed to depend entirely on having a family. Just like people who feel they would have better control of their lives with a slightly larger salary or who see a piece of clothing they have to have, my friend thought that something beyond herself could make her feel better about her life. She experienced desire.

Desire is wanting something from the world around us, and it is completely understandable why modern people experience this feeling. We are constantly bombarded with things that we are supposed to desire. We are surrounded by media conceived by people who are trying to sell us products and services. If you buy this makeup, you will be beautiful; if you go on this vacation, you will be able to recover from your crazy life; if you go to this college, you will land the career of your dreams. Even this book, *The One Plan,* was marketed to you as a promise: if you go through this program, you will live a better life. Each of these messages works to sell us on the idea that what we have is not enough— that consuming more, getting more, and having more is better than sticking with what we already have.

If getting $10,000 more a year could really give you complete control of your life, then there would be no problem if you suddenly had to spend $50,000 on an unexpected hospital visit. If the person who got the article of clothing could really experience total fulfillment from having it, they'd never need another article of clothing or anything else. And of course, though *The One Plan* may have been marketed to you in a way that suggests it will help you live a better life, it's not the book but practicing the methods that will ultimately lead you to let go of desire. If we really could take control of our lives like the promoters of these products and services are promising, we would have stopped needing new products and services long ago. We'd already feel fulfilled. Since we keep going out and buying more and more stuff, we are not.

The recurring theme in this struggle is that of expectations. When we desire something ("Ooh, that is the cutest dress!"), our minds tell us that we want it and we will be in a better situation when we get it. Desire creates an idea of what our lives will be like when we obtain whatever object, person, or situation we crave ("I will wear that dress, and I will be cute"). When we attach to this idea that something beyond ourselves will give us happiness, we create expectations.

My photographer friend had expectations that if she got married and had children, her life would finally have purpose. This meant that she was unhappy as a single woman without children, and changing this situation would make her happy. But what would happen if the husband she found, who at first glance was everything she thought she wanted, didn't entirely fulfill her expectations? If he is the reason she's happy, is he going to fulfill that role only if he meets certain conditions? What if he was initially a healthy, productive person who inspired her to live well, but five years into their marriage he encountered a professional setback and took to drinking and infidelity? Though few of us would encourage her to tolerate such behavior, my point is that when we expect something beyond ourselves to make us happy, we're guaranteeing that we won't ever be happy. In addition, we are placing an immense burden on our surroundings. People who marry someone who has such expectations have an even rougher time of it because of the burden they are given.

The fifth and final abstention, which we focused on in Weeks 9–10, was nongreed. This practice was based on letting go of what we already have to make room for what we need. The Yogic practice of contentment, known by the Sanskrit word *santosha,* is the flip side of this practice. Rather than overcoming the fear of not having enough, we're overcoming the desire to have more.

When Patanjali describes this practice in the Yoga Sutras, he says that when we experience contentment, we experience a state of supreme joy. When discussing the realm of the spirit in this book, we explored how each person has a spirit and that this part of ourselves is perfect, whole, and without want. Those who fully commit themselves to the Yogic path seek to realize this perfection during their time on earth. But this perfect entity can also be related to the practice of contentment. Since this tradition teaches us that each of us has a part of ourselves that's perfect, we don't ultimately need cute dresses, $10,000 raises, or even other people to feel whole. And because of the intensity of these desires, we've been unaware of a great secret: We already have everything we need to feel joyful. We already have ourselves.

A Perfect and Vital Reality

How will the practice of contentment take shape in your day-to-day life? For the second of Patanjali's five observations, your work will center on detaching from an object or a situation. Detachment is letting go of an object of desire and embracing the possibility that if you don't acquire this thing, something better will come your way. Whether you see a cute dress you would like to buy or you meet an ideal partner, you allow everything to happen exactly as it's supposed to. And as soon as you detach from something, you not only let go of desire but you allow unlimited abundance to come your way. Here is where you embrace the idea that you have everything you need to feel supreme joy.

If you experienced true contentment, you could put down this book and every other one and never have to buy or gather something to find fulfillment.

And when you do find something that makes you feel happy, you accept this as a new way to enrich the already perfect and vital reality of your existence.

The Body: Detachment from Things

The pursuit of contentment in the realm of the body relates to things we desire in the material world. When you feel contentment in this realm, you detach from possessions, food, and money. You may see something you'd like and buy it, but if you at some point don't have it anymore or it doesn't serve you in an ideal way, you will just as easily let it go. If you hear about a restaurant that serves the best food in town, you'll go and experience it for whatever it is and know that if your meal turns out to be a total dud, other good dining experiences are in your future. To pursue the physical realm of contentment does not equal not owning anything, nor does it mean that you won't ever want anything again. Feeling contentment in what you have means that you could either enjoy something you see or let it go and allow something else to come your way.

Contentment in the realm of the body looks like a person who has let go of much of what they had through their nongreed practice and is able to sustain this minimal way of life by not seeking to replace these things. When you are content with what you physically own and take into your body, you will accept that if you are supposed to have more, that will come to you as the world sees fit to provide it. If more does not come your way, that is also fine.

The Mind: Detachment from Circumstances

What if you decided it's time for you to change employers, and you learned of an opportunity that seems like your dream job? In this job, not only would you earn a larger salary, but you would have more responsibility, more interesting work to do, and a shorter commute. You get an interview, and the hiring manager who would be your boss is a lovely man who has interests similar to your own and seems like he'd be a tremendous source of encouragement and support. If you became attached to getting the job, you might think that this is the greatest professional opportunity you've ever had; if you don't get it, you'll be devastated and without any appealing options. When practicing contentment in the realm of the mind, however, we embrace the idea that the opportunities, situations, and circumstances that are presented to us can have as much false allure as an article of clothing. That so-called dream job isn't the thing you need in your life to be happy, nor is moving to the country or marrying the hottie you just met.

Again, this is not to say that you can't have the dream job, the life in the country, or the hottie. But instead of focusing solely on your desire, let go of those desires and leave the door open for even greater possibilities that you didn't even know existed. When you experience contentment in the mental realm of your practice, you will welcome all experiences that help you live a more enriched life—but will accept that other experiences may also hold that possibility for you.

The Spirit: Atop the Mountain

Imagine a man who goes to India to seek bliss. He finds a cave at the top of a mountain, lives in that cave, tends to a small garden where he grows his food, and does little else but sit in quiet contemplation. He is peaceful and content with the little he has. Now, imagine this same man plucked from his cave, flown around the world, and placed on a square of concrete in the middle of the intersection of W. 45th Street, 7th Avenue, and Broadway in New York City—in the middle of Times Square. There is no soil here, so he can't grow a garden. There are no caves, save for the nearby entrance to the 42nd Street subway station—and that particular cave is overrun with people. And there won't ever be quiet, for of all of the neighborhoods of this enormous city, Times Square is the one that truly never sleeps. This man experienced peace, contentment, and joy when he lived in his cave atop a mountain in India. If he feels that same contentment in the densest, most material version of Western society, then he truly lives in the realm of his perfect spirit. He has attained supreme joy.

When you exist in contentment within the realm of the spirit, you enjoy the endless bounty of brilliance to be found within. Just as practicing nongreed allows room for abundance, practicing contentment in this highest realm allows for everything in the universe to come to you in as perfect a form as it can.

The Plan

Practicing contentment is ambitious, because in the modern world we are inundated with stimulation of every kind. Considering that there are many opportunities to indulge our desires and that letting go of expectations is a struggle in any time period, the contentment practices provided for you in the One Plan will be fairly straightforward exercises.

The Realm of the Body

You will benefit from practicing contentment in the realm of the body if you buy a lot of things for yourself, if your response to a really bad day is to go on a shopping spree or indulge in pampering services, if you particularly look forward to mealtime, if you're particularly frustrated by money and don't feel you have enough of it, and if you believe physical things will make you happier.

Your task for these two weeks is to eat your lunch in silence. Though you may often eat with coworkers or friends, at your desk browsing the Internet, while using your phone to send e-mails and text messages, while reading books or periodicals, or even while zoning out in front of the TV, for these two weeks you will do nothing but focus on eating. It can seem boring and even off-putting to not distract yourself with activities, but craving distraction is a form of discontentment. Eating in silence allows for greater appreciation of the food available to us and gives us an opportunity to take in our surroundings without needing to control them. In training yourself to be content with the simple act of eating, you will learn that you don't require more and more things to be happy.

If you are with other people during these two weeks, let them know that you are practicing in this way and invite them to join you in eating in silence together. Beyond these two weeks, arrange to eat your lunch in silence at least once a week to train yourself to not crave more interaction with your physical surroundings.

The Realm of the Mind

You will benefit from exploring the mental realm of contentment if you have succeeded in working past your attachment to objects and other material things and are able to live a minimalistic lifestyle. You no longer appease yourself with shopping sprees or lavish meals. You no longer feel compelled to have money to be happy. Most of us struggle a great deal to embody the physical realm of contentment in our behaviors, so you are absolutely serving yourself to remain focused on these elements of your life for as long as you need to. If, however, you feel you have worked past these attachments, then it is time for your work to focus on the mental realm of contentment.

Discontentment takes place in the realm of the mind when we seek a specific situation or circumstance as a source of happiness—much like my photographer friend did when she based her happiness on finding a husband. We begin to practice contentment when we let go of a particular situation and embrace the idea that not experiencing it may allow another, more ideal situation to present itself. If my photographer friend were to not get married, she could do something else, like spend years traveling the world and seeing things that most other people will never see.

Over these two weeks, your task is to come up with a situation or circumstance you desire in seven different areas of your life (recreational, comfort-based, domestic, platonic, professional, romantic, and familial). You will spend two days with each desire. On the first day, you will think of a desire you have in the area assigned to that day and consider things you could do instead. Then, on the second day, you are to take a single step toward that alternate possibility. Though you might not pursue any further steps, the point of the exercise is to create a new reality in your mind that helps you let go of the desire. For example, on Days 11 and 12 of these two weeks, you are to focus on the romantic aspect of your life. You might desire someone you're communicating with online, but are not sure if they're going to reciprocate your interest. On Day 11, you would identify this desire and consider an alternate situation—perhaps communication with someone different or letting go of the person completely. On Day 12, you would take a step toward communicating with someone else you imagine wanting to meet. By investing even a small amount of time and energy in a different reality, you are letting go of the idea that the first person is necessary for you to be happy. This will lessen your attachment to finding someone and emphasize that you don't need anyone but yourself to be content. Once you've practiced contentment, you will attract someone who is also content if you are supposed to be with someone. Practice in these seven areas during these two weeks using the following structure:

- DAYS 1–2: *Identify and take one step toward detaching from a recreational desire.* This could be going to a ball game, to see a movie, to a concert, to a casino, or another outlet. Consider what you desire, and find another activity that you could enjoy instead.

- DAYS 3–4: *Identify and take one step toward detaching from a comfort-based desire.* This could be receiving a massage, going on a vacation, or receiving another sort of pampering experience. Consider what you desire, and find an alternate way to spend your time that might afford you enjoyment without indulging in the same way.

- DAYS 5–6: *Identify and take one step toward detaching from a domestic desire.* This could be owning a home, getting a specific dream home, getting a second home, expanding your current home, refurnishing your home, or some other desire for more than what you currently have. If you're fixated on acquiring a specific home, consider what other space you might benefit from living in. If you simply desire to own something for the sake of owning it, consider other things you might be able to build with your resources (for instance, travel opportunities or charitable work).

- DAYS 7–8: *Identify and take one step toward detaching from a platonic desire.* You may find that you desire to spend time with someone you consider a friend but who either isn't available or doesn't reciprocate your interest. Consider a different person you might befriend instead.

- DAYS 9–10: *Identify and take one step toward detaching from a professional desire.* You may covet a specific job or just one that's different from the one you currently have. Consider a different opportunity that might be available to you, be it finding a new way to enjoy your current job or creating one for yourself.

- DAYS 11–12: *Identify and take one step toward detaching from a romantic desire.* If you are single, there might be someone you wish to be with, or you might not have a specific idea but wish to be with someone all the same. If you're in a relationship, you might wish for it to be more than what it is. If you're single, consider how you might spend time doing something you can't do if you're in a relationship, and if you're in a relationship, find a way to initiate something new between the two of you.

- DAYS 13–14: *Identify and take one step toward detaching from a familial desire.* You may yearn for children, wish you had had them though it's too late, or wish that the children or other family members you do have behaved differently. If you are childless, consider what opportunities you may create because you don't have children. If you have children, find a new way to give your time to them without living through them or expecting anything in return.

When we feel discontentment about our situation in life, tension often builds up. You may experience tension when you examine your desires. Each time you have a thought that creates this feeling, simply observe which aspect of it annoys you. Identify the nature of the desire that you are trying to fulfill. As you move on beyond these two weeks, you will start to become more aware of your desires and the expectations you are building in your mind. Eventually, the desires will also be gone.

The Realm of the Spirit

When we pursue a spiritual path such as the one outlined in this program, we can become committed to it and its various methods to the point of becoming attached—in a sense, we become attached to being detached. The person who goes off to a place like India and holes up on a mountaintop has committed himself or herself to working in the realm of the mind; in some way, that person is attached to practicing detachment. When you can let go of the mountain or another supposedly peaceful situation and experience serenity and happiness wherever you are and while doing whatever you are doing, then you have truly realized the contentment born from perfection of the spirit.

You will discover a peaceful mountain in your contentment practice when you experience joyful peace in all endeavors you participate in. If you can enter a relationship without expectations, look at that relationship as simply an opportunity to serve the other person, and adore the perfect lessons you learn in being with that person, then you are practicing contentment in the realm of the spirit. To begin this practice, let go of any exercise or question regarding your contentment and leave all expectations alone. Become an observer of everything. Walk with the body, witness with the mind, and let the Spirit act through you.

Emerging as a Masterpiece

As you move forward in your pursuit of the observations in this program, you will begin to make greater time commitments on a day-to-day basis. Though you will be spending more time with this work, you will find greater focus and enrichment in all aspects of your day—and your improved focus will likely allow you to get things done more thoroughly. With practices like contentment, you may experience results that are less immediate than, say, the freedom of removing clutter through nongreed practices or the moisturized feeling you get from oiling your nose. You are taking far more refined steps in chipping away at the marble—you're not knocking off such large chunks anymore. But just because a stroke is more subtle doesn't mean that it's less important.

Putting It Together

If you are pursuing this program entirely in the realm of the body, your routine will be as follows:

- Continue your daily purity practices each morning.

- Take herbal tea twice a day to continue building strength and cleanliness.

- Eat your lunch in silence for these two weeks.

And remember . . .

- Continue eating half as much processed food and unhealthy substances as you did before, avoid eating during the last two hours of the day, and release your sexual essence half as often as you did before Week 7. Avoid accumulating more possessions.

- Continue building your nonviolence, truthfulness, and nonstealing behaviors to the best of your ability. Continue participating in a physical activity that requires presence of mind at least once every two weeks.

If you are practicing exclusively in the realm of the mind, your daily practice over these two weeks will look like this:

- Continue practicing the Gayatri Mantra each morning.

- Practice exploring detachment from a desire in each of the seven categories outlined earlier.

And remember . . .

- Continue eating natural foods, avoid eating in the last five hours of the day and after 7 P.M., and continue to have sex in moderation.

- Continue your nonviolence, truthfulness, and nonstealing practices, and avoid sexual thoughts. Continue to let go of attachments to people and situations that you are keeping out of fear.

burnt out, but in a good way

AUSTERITY

N THE FALL OF 2009, WHEN I TRAVELED TO INDIA TO STUDY WITH MY TEACHER and take one of my customary journeys, I invited my friend Neil to join me. He and I had collaborated on various projects, and he was also developing a self-realization practice. I wanted to document the trip for my website, books, and coaching, and I knew he'd be helpful with that task. We traveled around India for two months visiting temples, ashrams, and holy places to explore our practices in new and more involved ways.

When I was a fashion model, I was exposed to many people around the world. I often spent time with models who were supercharged with sexual energy. Most of them welcomed the attention they typically received, and that attention often became palpable. After all, what nineteen-year-old could say no to all that attention? I could be walking down the street alongside a fellow model, and the vibe would suddenly change. Without anyone saying anything, I knew there was a man or woman stalking us—as if we were being hunted.

It was after Neil and I had been traveling together for several weeks that I discovered he was a hunter. We would be walking through a town, and suddenly the vibe would change. We would be talking about a temple we had visited, an Ayurvedic treatment we had observed, or some other feature of our travels, and I would realize that Neil wasn't thinking about any of these things anymore. I would stop walking to look at Neil, and sure enough, he'd be eyeing his next conquest: a beautiful, curvaceous serving of Indian cuisine.

Rather than being on the hunt for sexual conquests, Neil was on the hunt for food. A lot of the time I spent traveling with Neil was defined by whether he would be able to feed himself in what he considered a satisfying way. His mood was always heavy until he got something to eat. He didn't want to eat at eight o'clock at night, like most of India does, so he was often left with random snacks sold at carts alongside whatever road we were walking along at his preferred dinnertime of 6 P.M. When I teased him about it, he mumbled something about not being able to help being raised in a Jewish American household. According to him, this made it impossible to not obsess over food.

I could have predicted Neil's reaction to fasting for ten days. Though we spent much of the two months looking for places to explore our practices, I wanted to spend a couple of stationary weeks committed to silence and an absence of food. The practice would be to push ourselves out of our comfort zones and see if any burdensome thoughts might unravel and be addressed in a productive way. When we arrived in Kankhal, a small town in northwestern India, I declared this was where we would explore this work. Neil didn't have much to say in response—though I gathered from what seemed like a returning heaviness in his mood that he had a few thoughts about what was to come.

But we were both committed to our path and moved forward with the plan. Neil only made it through six days of fasting instead of ten. Following the end of the fast, his hunt for food became even more intense. He told me that he believed his need to satisfy his hunger made perfect sense, given how malnourished his body had become.

We left Kankhal after about two weeks to visit Varanasi, a major hub of spiritual growth and activity in northern India. Recently, it has become a touristy place, though much of its spiritual significance is preserved by local sages hidden to the untrained eye. When Neil and I were there, we were approached by a constant flurry of people attempting to sell us food products, silk items, and motorized or bicycle-based rickshaw rides. Either Neil or I would decline. When they insisted, Neil would be firmer: "We told you *no*." When they still persisted, he would say, "No! Get away. *Now!*" Neil struggled as a traveler, but now he had reached his limit. Because of his culture shock, his desire to compensate for the fast, and what sounded like a deep-seated hatred of every salesperson who approached us, he went on a tirade about how certain people in his life seemed to always make him feel guilty about things that he felt were out of his control.

"It's like no matter what I do," he said through gnashed teeth, "nothing's ever good enough for them. I try to be a good friend or family member, I try to listen to their problems, and then I have to endure them complaining about how I haven't called often enough, or they start volunteering information about what they think of my life without my even asking for their opinion. Screw them. Screw them all."

He said all of this—as well as a few choice swear words—as we were sitting in one of the rickshaws we actually did hire after being approached by its driver. I had to admit that I didn't really know what he was talking about in the moment; he just seemed to need to spew out poison, and I wanted him to feel free to do so. But later in our trip I discovered that in that moment Neil had started to realize that he had been defining relationships by his ability to keep the other person happy. He would address what the other person wanted at the expense of what he wanted for himself. It might seem random that he was confronting aggressive silk vendors one minute and making poisonous statements about his entire life the next, but in the days that followed I started to notice a shift. Angry as that outburst was, he no longer seemed as heavy. He was still on the hunt for food, but when I asked him about what he had said on that rickshaw, he gave me an apologetic look. "When I go back to the States," he said, "I'm still going to try to serve my friends and family. But I'll work to always serve myself as well."

Leaving Nothing but Embers

There are many situations in life in which we feel discomfort. We might feel too cold if the temperature unexpectedly drops, or we might feel too hot if the air conditioner breaks. We might feel isolated and lonely if we're stuck in a hotel room far from home, or we might feel starved if we haven't eaten all day. Throughout such seemingly adverse situations, we might feel upset or frustrated. Then, when we're no longer cold, hot, isolated, or hungry, we're ready to accept that though discomfort does happen, the only thing we can do is get out of it as quickly as possible.

Now, let's say you live in a house and it's the middle of winter. What is the difference between a fire caused by an electrical problem in the basement and a fire that you light in a wood-burning stove? This might seem like a silly question, for one fire is a safe, contained way to keep the house warm, and the other fire is a hazardous situation that could burn the entire house to the ground. One fire keeps the harsh winter away, and the other might put you suddenly in the middle of that harshness—probably without a coat or proper shoes. But the difference between these two fires is like the difference between experiencing discomfort and wanting it to end as quickly as possible, and experiencing it as the next observation outlined by Patanjali: austerity, or *tapas*.

The essential difference between the two fires is that one, as an accident, has tremendous destructive potential, and the other, as a deliberate effort, serves a function. Discomfort, like fire, can be destructive when it gets out of control, but it can also be used as a tool. Austerity is seeking out discomfort for the sake of personal growth. Just as we use fire to burn wood in a stove, we use discomfort to burn off physical and mental toxins. In fact, the literal translation of the word *tapas* is "heat."

But how can discomfort help us grow? Neil and I were practicing austerity when we fasted and observed silence in India. We said to ourselves, "I'm going to not eat or talk for days at a time, and in doing so I will purge myself of the toxins in my body and mind." What happened to Neil is what often happens to people who go on fasts or engage in other practices that lead to intense discomfort: he hit an emotional wall. To continue on with his life, he had to find a way over, around, or through it. His whole world unraveled before him, and he suddenly saw something that he hadn't seen previously. When he burned off the toxins in his stomach and mind, he was left with only a few embers of the tension and anger he had been holding on to. The fast allowed the physical purge, and then the episode on the rickshaw served as a way for him to clear himself of the mental struggles that had boiled to the surface. Neil was so much lighter and less burdened afterward that he was almost like a different person. He fasted for six days, but he unearthed several decades.

Practicing austerity can take many forms, and it can happen with different intentions. Other aspects of Patanjali's abstentions and observations, such as continence and purity, are also forms of austerity. But whatever the intention, this tool can be of tremendous benefit to those seeking greater happiness through the Yogic path; it allows us to overcome obstacles, work past physical and mental burdens, and ultimately completely let go of stored-up pain or tension.

The Useful Side of Discomfort

When practicing austerity, it's important to take small steps. When Neil and I fasted, we had already been practicing various aspects of Yoga for some time. This gave us the grounding to work through difficulties in a productive way. When pursuing this work, we can experience a lot of frustration. It can therefore be difficult to determine if the challenges that come up are productive or not. With the help of the body/mind/spirit structure, however, you will be able to give yourself the most beneficial challenges to overcome for wherever you are in your austerity practice. Below is an overview of how this practice may be pursued through the three realms.

The Body: A Physical Burn

Austerity, in its most basic form, involves taking on physical discomfort to purge toxins from the body. The most obvious way to do this is through fasting. When the body no longer has food to digest, it moves on to toxins that have built up. After the fast, the body has a lightness from having purged itself of its burdens—perhaps chemicals accumulated from unnatural foods, or simply the substances that come from life in our modern world. Refraining from speaking (taking a vow of silence) can serve a similar function. Given how much we rely on verbal communication with others in our day-to-day lives, not speaking certainly causes discomfort and can lead to greater self-understanding. Other ways of practicing physical austerity include putting ourselves in an uncomfortable environment for extended periods of time or avoiding gratifying activities like sex.

While engaging in austerity, your work is to persevere. During a fast, you might think to yourself, "Man, I really want something to eat right now." If you ate food as soon as you started to feel the pangs of hunger, you would no longer be creating an opportunity to purge yourself. When you feel hunger, you then think, "This is good for me, and there will be food again tomorrow. For now, I will continue on." As things get harder, they also help us become more powerful. At the end, the body will have burned off some toxicity, and you'll be healthier for it.

The Mind: A Mental Burn

You may have noticed in the story about Neil that he put himself through a physical form of austerity by avoiding eating, but his purge on the rickshaw involved how he felt about relationships back home—his mental condition. Because of the close connection between body and mind, physical purges and mental purges often blur together as one affects the other. I once fasted for twenty-eight days to break a mental habit regarding relationships. Physical austerity can have a mental impact on our lives, but there are also specifically mental practices.

Whereas physical austerity relates to what goes into our bodies, mental austerity relates to what goes into our minds. Mental austerity calls on us to use seemingly negative stimulation that comes our way as a way to burn off toxic thoughts. If a person spewed out a particularly nasty, hateful insult at you, you would probably react strongly, right? You might insult the person right back, or you might break down in tears. But if you were practicing austerity in the realm of the mind, you would look at each insult thrown at you, each comment that you disagree with, and every other form of problematic mental stimulation as a chance to burn off mental toxins. Someone could come up to you and say that you were an idiot, and you would take it in as a gift. They would be helping you know what your practice is in that moment.

Eventually, when you've accepted all the negative stimulation around you and burned off your toxins, your mind will be as light as a stomach that hasn't been filled in days.

The Spirit: A Light Emerges

In the introduction, I mentioned my friend and mentor Ron, who introduced me to this path before he died of AIDS in 2000. Ron lived with HIV for many years, but there is something about his life that is even more inspirational. Even though his body was broken and he was so weak in the final months that he could barely move, he didn't live with the heavy burden of one whose time on earth was slipping away. He had let go of attachment to his body, because he understood that regardless of his physical state, his spirit remained pure and perfectly intact. In the final days I spent with him, he was full of light.

You will know that you are ready to explore austerity in the realm of the spirit when you see yourself and everything else as one entity. When exploring austerity in this realm, our work is to accept and embrace our situations in life—no matter how broken, diseased, downtrodden, or oppressed they have become. Because our spirits are already perfect, we allow this perfection to guide us in helping others. When others live with illness, we provide support. When others are downtrodden, we give them our shoulders to lean on. When others turn their hurt against us to bend us to their will, we offer them more than just gratitude for the opportunity to practice—we offer them our love.

The Plan

Though there are many ways we can burn off physical and mental toxins, the One Plan provides a few simple exercises in which to explore this practice. But remember, just because they're simple, it doesn't mean they're easy.

The Realm of the Body

You will benefit from exploring austerity in the realm of the body if you've never fasted and find the idea particularly intimidating. To begin your work with austerity, your task for the first thirteen days of this part of the program is to go on a brisk walk for fifteen or twenty minutes each day or, if you prefer, go for a light jog (be sure to stretch before and after and wear enough clothing to induce a sweat). You could spend this time in a steam tent if you have access to one; look online for sources. Any of these activities will help you burn off physical toxins. Though walking or jogging may seem like little more than light exercise, setting an intention to practice austerity means that you will have greater awareness of what—if anything—comes up in the process. If something particularly poignant or daunting comes up for you through these activities, simply observe it and take note of when it comes up again.

On Day 14 you are to conduct your first twenty-four-hour fast. Starting when you wake up, take in nothing but warm water throughout the day. Keep a container with you if you're out and about, but abstain from eating or drinking anything other than water—even herbal tea. Continue straight through to bedtime. When you wake up the next morning, resume your regular diet. Many feelings of discomfort or frustration will likely come up for you in the course of this day. Allow yourself to have these feelings. This is your body digesting the toxic substances inside.

The Realm of the Mind

Your work with austerity in the realm of the mind is twofold: you will practice a lengthier fast, and you will use the Presence Practice to burn off mental toxicity. For the fast, choose any three days in each of the two weeks devoted to austerity, for a total of six days. You may decide to fast one day and eat the next, alternating back and forth throughout the two weeks. Or you may decide to fast three days and then eat for four days. However you configure this work, be sure to remain true to your commitment. The intense fast will help you burn off physical toxins, but you will also likely hit a wall similar to the one Neil experienced in India, and this will help you shift your mind.

- If you fast for one day and eat the next, eat normally but be sure to have a cup of hot water at least an hour before you resume eating.

- If you fast for two days straight, resume eating by drinking some hot water, and then a little overcooked rice or vegetable soup one hour later as your first meal. Then resume normal eating after two hours.

- If you fast for three days straight, resume eating by taking some hot water, having a bland cup of vegetable broth with a pinch of black pepper and ginger an hour later, and again taking vegetable broth half a day later before eating solids. Avoid raw foods on the first day after fasting.

Your other task for these two weeks is to use the Presence Practice to remind yourself to accept abuse from others. People may say insensitive, cutting, or even outright mean things to you to which you might react with strong, contrary emotions. While sitting for five minutes, ask yourself the following questions:

- When someone is unpleasant or nasty to me, am I prone to retaliate with aggression?

- Do I retaliate by playing the wounded victim?

- Do I break down in tears?

- Do I take the abuse in the moment but then say nasty things about the person behind his or her back?

- Do I take the abuse in the moment but then get down on myself for being inadequate?

- Do I have violent thoughts toward the person?

- Do I have vengeful thoughts?

Then, when someone does act abusively toward you, remind yourself that this is an opportunity to burn off the toxicity in your mind, and accept it as a gift. When you succeed in doing this, you might even see a shift in the other person's energy.

The Realm of the Spirit

Work with austerity in the realm of the spirit can become intense. This intensity may be fueled by a debilitating illness, a significant loss, or some other source of significant pain and suffering. Ron told me that his mind was not glad to have HIV, but the disease saved his spirit from having to suffer in a body ever again.

If you, like Ron, suffer from some debilitating disease, your work during these two weeks is to spend some time deciding how best to move forward in relation to it. Would working to resolve the illness come from a determination to fulfill a specific purpose, or would it come from a place of fear for dying? For example, if you have heart disease, your practice would be to decide whether to have a heart transplant. Not having it may open you up to experiencing peace and contentment during your remaining time on earth and letting go of your fears. In this realm, there is no fear, but guidance to do what the Spirit wills.

If you don't have any disease, your task is to put yourself in a situation of all-encompassing, useful discomfort, perhaps serving others who are sick or finding other ways to experience your purpose, be it in an isolated environment or with others. Because of all of the austerity practices you've already done in previous years, you will know what your work must be in this realm. You must then use these circumstances to work past whatever fear you have of the point in time when you finally pass on and attain ultimate community with the Spirit.

Emerging as a Masterpiece

Your work during these two weeks devoted to austerity will add a little time to your daily routine, but some of the work, such as fasting, will be less labor intensive and more, well, labored. During your fast, you may feel particularly put off by the discomfort you're feeling. This is perfectly okay, even expected. The struggle is simply the austerity work doing its job, and this difficulty will absolutely make you stronger.

Putting It Together

If you are pursuing this program entirely within the realm of the body, your routine will be as follows:

- Continue your daily purity practices.

- Take herbal tea twice a day to continue building strength and cleanliness.

- Continue to eat your lunch in silence at least once a week.

- Go for a brief walk or jog each day, or sit in a steam tent.

- Fast on the fourteenth day.

And remember . . .

- Continue eating half as much processed food and unhealthy substances as you did previously, avoid eating during the last two hours of the day, and release your sexual essence half as often as you did before Week 7. Continue to avoid accumulating more possessions.

- Continue building your nonviolence, truthfulness, and nonstealing behaviors to the best of your ability. Continue participating in a physical activity that requires presence of mind at least once every two weeks.

If you are practicing exclusively within the realm of the mind, your daily practice over these two weeks will look like this:

- Spend five minutes in the morning using your Presence Practice to focus on accepting insulting situations as an opportunity to burn off mental toxins.

- Spend ten minutes of your morning repeating the Gayatri Mantra.

- Fast for three days of each week devoted to austerity.

And remember . . .

- Continue eating natural foods, refraining from eating during the last five hours of the day and after 7 P.M., and having sex in moderation.

- Continue your nonviolence, truthfulness, and nonstealing practices, and continue avoiding sexual thoughts. Continue to let go of attachments to people and situations that you are keeping out of fear.

- Continue to take note of your situational desires and create alternate possibilities for your life.

removing the layers of dust

SELF-STUDY

TRAVELED TO INDIA IN 2009 PARTLY TO FIND A NEW TEACHER. THOUGH I HAD learned a great deal from my guru Vasudevan at Arsha Yoga, we focused mainly on my development as an Ayurveda therapist. I wanted to be initiated into a practice more centered on the Yogic path. When I visited Arsha in 2009, I purchased a copy of the Bhagavad Gita from the bookstore. As I began reading the ancient text and its accompanying commentary, I discovered I had found a way to broaden my exploration of the Yogic path.

About a month later, I was staying in a small town outside of Haridwar. One day, out of nowhere, I was approached by a man on the street. He told me in perfect English that if I needed anything during my stay, just to let him know. I wasn't sure why, but I decided that I needed to talk to him.

"I'm here to look for a teacher," I said to him.

"Oh yes?" said the man. "Then I would like you to come with me to see my teacher tomorrow."

"What does he teach?" I asked him.

"He teaches the Bhagavad Gita."

The following morning I joined my new friend, Deva. We walked about twenty minutes from the ashram I was staying at to visit another ashram. It was situated on a large, open road near the Ganges River amid a scattering of other buildings. As Deva and I walked through the ashram, he explained that the teacher was born into a wealthy family but then cast it all aside to follow his guru and study the Gita and that he now lived in a small room in this ashram. Deva led me to a door at the end of a small building.

When we walked inside, I was greeted by the enormous smile of one of the oldest men I'd ever seen. He was a thin little man who wore a *dhoti* wrapped around his legs. He wore great big glasses as he read from a large book that looked as old as he did. I found out later that he was nearly a hundred years old. Having committed nearly eighty years to this work, this man radiated peace and purpose. Many years ago, he had assisted his guru in translating another edition of the Gita.

My new friend and I were alone in the room with him that day, and he began the lesson by reading from the book. After he read from a passage, he divulged not just the translation but the hidden meaning of the words. At the end of his talk, he welcomed questions.

"How must you practice if you don't have a teacher?" I asked.

"The Gita is like a dusty glass-top coffee table," he said in clear English. "If you don't have a teacher in the physical world, you must keep reading the same material over and over again, and your inner guru will translate. Each time you read it, you remove a layer of dust. With dedication, patience, and discipline, you'll eventually remove all the dust and see right through the glass."

He explained that reading the Gita, like any form of self-study, reflects what we already know at the spirit level. When we pursue this work on ourselves, we are eventually guided by the great knower of all that sits inside.

Eventually, our class came to an end, and I thanked the teacher for his time. As Deva and I walked back to my ashram, I marveled at how nothing in life is ever a coincidence. I had wanted to start learning about the Gita, and here was one of the original translators of a still available version of it. I had found the teacher I was seeking—but now I needed to pursue the guru within.

The Circular Life

All of us have had to struggle through adversity. Sometimes those struggles arrive because of a troubled situation, a disappointing experience, or something someone did or said that we just didn't like. In response, we get upset, wonder why such a bad thing happened to us, and complain about it to anyone who will listen until we think we feel better, store away the negative feelings, and then allow those feelings to surface when something triggers them. Then, if one of these obstacles makes a repeat appearance, we think, why did such a bad thing happen to me . . . *again?* We experience what we perceive as more negative feelings, and the cycle continues.

This is what I call the circular life. When we experience situations that we perceive as adversity, our egos want to control them. But since we cannot control the outside world, the ego can only manipulate our perception of it, so we have the *illusion* of control. Maybe you are prone to overeat, and have been since you were very young. To assume control, your ego says, "I keep eating like this because I'm constantly bombarded with commercials and advertisements enticing me to eat fast food." The ego says you are struggling in your eating habits because of the advertisers. However, plenty of other people see the same advertisements but don't overeat. Some even avoid that type of food because of the advertisements. If you've been overeating all your life, it likely involves a deep-seated issue in need of resolution. By allowing the ego to tell this story, you are neglecting to identify the root cause of why you are continually overeating. Rather than observing the pattern and determining when it started, you are piling layer after layer of dust over the simple truth of your own spirit. In covering the spirit with more and more layers of dust, we perpetuate struggle and suffering.

When I asked the guru how to study the Gita without a teacher, he said that continual reading would enable me to see its basic truth. Much like the Yoga Sutras, the Bhagavad Gita was written by sages who embodied self-realization. Through their devotion to their practice, they reflected the spirit in much of their earthly experience. When they came to a place of oneness, they wrote the Bhagavad Gita. In a sense, they took down spiritual dictation. I was instructed by the guru to continue reading the Gita so that I would eventually uncover its meaning. I would eliminate the layers of dust until they were all gone. Under this dust would be a divine light that had been dictated for me by the sages.

The next of Patanjali's observations is self-study, or *svadhyaya*. This practice calls on us to study our bodies and minds so that we may ultimately gain knowledge of who we truly are. As living beings, we are each born from the Spirit and therefore embody this perfection within. But when we're stuck in a circular life, we continually encounter circumstances that upset us, people we find hurtful or antagonizing, and any number of other situations that we suffer through again and again. But since each of us is of the Spirit and contains a divine light within, we can move beyond the circular life, gradually remove each layer of dust, and ultimately reveal that light. With this light, we find the purpose of our lives.

When those of us living in the West go about changing our lives, we typically do so in a logical way. We impose the mind onto the situation by analyzing it. We might deduce that we're inadequate ("I look disgusting, therefore I should go on a diet") or that we aren't living up to an idea of what we've set out to be ("I'm supposed to be a yogi, so I shouldn't be eating like this"). However, imposing the mind on a situation—"I should, I shouldn't, I'm supposed to"—continues its circular workings. Even if we do create change, we're doing so from a place of ego. This perpetuates limited amounts of change and much more suffering.

In contrast, the Yogic path teaches us to observe. We do this by continually tuning in to our bodies and minds so that new knowledge or information emerges through intuition. Self-study uses observation to clear away the dust and see the fundamental truth about ourselves. If we attempted to answer the question, "Am I eating the right food?" we would read article after article, measure all sorts of numbers pertaining to our diet (calories, fat, etc.) and our physical health (blood pressure, cholesterol, etc.), and then deduce what we should and shouldn't eat. If we sought to explore this question intuitively, we would pose it to ourselves, let go of a need for an answer in any specific moment, experiment with different food choices, and then see how we feel over time. In letting go of a need for specific conclusions ("I weigh ten more pounds than my doctor says I'm supposed to, so I'm going to eat only salads"), we allow room for discoveries ("I've been eating dinners of cooked vegetables for several months, and I feel great").

When we use our intuition, we call on the perfect truth that exists within to help us create shifts. Analysis relies on imposing the mind ("Everyone else goes to college at eighteen, so the fact that I'm thirty-five means I'm too old"), but our intuitive process relies on the fundamental truth of the perfect spirit ("In this moment, my purpose is to become a nurse, and I need to go to college to do so—regardless of my age"). Through observation, we become aware of the situation we are in and how that situation may be significant, but we don't impose our insecurities, attachments, or other products of the ego onto it. By observing ourselves, we become aware of what we need to attain greater balance. We eat certain things because we feel healthy when we eat them. We go to school to study nursing because that is what we must do to be a nurse. We leave the door open to all possibilities so we can choose from an unlimited source.

Lexie, a client I worked with on my show, experienced significant stress. One therapy I suggested was to paint her cold, gray wall a warm yellow that was more conducive to calmness and meditation. She said she knew when she painted the wall gray that it was the wrong color, but she still allowed the idea in her mind—that gray was more "stylish"—to form the basis of her aesthetic decision. She knew from a more intuitive source that the wall needed to be something different, but she chose to ignore it and let her actions be dictated by her mind. And when I ruined the gray wall by painting "paint me" in yellow, her mind dictated that she try to strangle me.

Making decisions and taking action based on our intuitive source helps us move beyond the limitations our minds have imposed through tradition, religion, and society and create a sense of balance. This balance forms the basis of how we evolve through our practice of self-study.

Removing the Dust

During my modeling days, I had a very relaxed schedule. I went to bed late and woke up late on days I wasn't working. Once I started learning about the Yogic path, I read about how important it was to go to bed early and wake up early. I had it in my head that I wanted to live a more spiritual life and thought if I changed my sleeping routine I would better fulfill this idea of being "more spiritual." But I didn't have any success in going to bed early or waking up early. I continued to crawl out of bed late and with just as much lethargy. As I immersed myself further in this path over many years, though, I noticed that when I did have to wake up earlier I felt invigorated and ready to pursue my day with far greater energy. I realized that getting up early wasn't a way to be more spiritual, but it did have a fundamentally positive effect on my life. I then decided that I needed to start getting up early, and even though I was inconsistent at first, I finally trained myself to get up early. Productivity thrived.

This was a simple way of practicing self-study. Early on, my ego was attached to the idea of a spiritual lifestyle, and therefore I was trying to change my life through analysis ("If I get up early, I'll be more spiritual"). But when I simply observed the benefits of getting up early, I felt a greater sense of purpose in pursuing that as a regular habit. Waking up early didn't make me more spiritual, but it gave me more time and energy to practice my spiritual path. I realized through intuition that I was perpetuating an unwanted pattern and adjusted my behavior. Though self-study centers on observing a situation and building awareness of it, the final part of this process, creating change, can be explored in different ways in the realms of the body, mind, and spirit. But regardless of which realm we work in, creating change is based on a simple concept: take action from a place of observation and acceptance, not analysis and conclusions.

The Body: Clearing Away Physical Dust

Ayurvedic tradition teaches that each person is born into this world with a basic physical nature. We inherit this nature from our parents, much like we inherit our facial features or our hair color. As natural, organic beings, we are a product of the five elements: fire, water, earth, air, and ether. Some people have more earthy energy, and therefore may, like me, be challenged by lethargy, while others have more fiery energy, making them prone to anger and intensity. Though each person has a different combination of these energies at any given moment, when we're born into the world, we have a basic, almost default-like nature that we call *prakruti*. Just as we are genetically predisposed to have a certain look or hair color, we're also predisposed to have a particular energy in our bodies. Though our energy can shift over time, this basic nature determines the diseases we're prone to and the methods we must use to keep our bodies in balance.

The ancient sages who developed Ayurvedic medicine determined that we combine the five elements in nature into three energy types, known as *doshas*.

- The *Vata* dosha is a combination of the air and ether elements. It is responsible for all movement. Just as blowing air on hanging clothes helps the clothes dry, Vata energy dries the body. People who have too much Vata energy are prone to constipation (lack of moisture and movement in the gastrointestinal tract) and anxiety (too much movement in the brain), among other conditions.

- The *Pitta* dosha is a combination of the fire and water elements. Just as touching fire to a piece of paper will burn up the paper, the body burns out from too much Pitta energy. People who have too much Pitta energy are prone to digestive disorders like hyperacidity (too much heat in the stomach), and irritations of the skin (too much heat escaping from the stomach).

- The *Kapha* dosha is a combination of the earth and water elements. Just as dousing a flower with too much water and dirt can overwhelm it, too much Kapha energy encumbers the body. People who have too much Kapha energy are prone to respiratory disorders (too much moisture in the lungs) and lethargy (too much heaviness in the body because of mucus and other impurities), as well as other forms of encumbrance.

Though we have all three energy types in our bodies, we have different ratios, and this makes us vulnerable to imbalances: for example, if the Pitta energy becomes too intense, the body undergoes excessive metabolization and produces excessive heat, leading to illness and disease. When we determine what our ratio is and how it may be out of balance, we're able to make better decisions about how we eat and craft a beneficial lifestyle.

Ayurvedic doctors and practitioners go through an extensive process to determine the relative balance of a patient's doshas. From there we are able to determine the underlying causes of the patients' illnesses and what they can do to avoid illness. We use the outside of the body as a map to determine what is happening on the inside. If a patient's skin is dry, it is likely that the Vata energy is out of balance. We also use what is happening on the inside the body—pain, discomfort, or even symptoms—to make similar observations. Then we are able to treat the patient in a way that emulates self-study: after observing and becoming aware of the patient's imbalances, we create change by having the patient do the opposite of what caused the imbalance. If they have too much Vata energy, we help them reduce dryness in the body. If they have too much Pitta energy, we help them reduce heat. If they have too much Kapha energy, we help them reduce moisture. The best Ayurvedic doctors and practitioners don't make a determination about their patient's prakruti in the first couple of sessions, for making intuitive assessments—removing the dust covering up their patient's condition—takes time.

Through the One Plan, you'll learn to observe your body as well as your dosha type. With greater knowledge of our basic physical nature and the relative balances or imbalances of the body at any given time, we're able to create change as necessary. When we create this type of change, we create peace in the physical realm.

The Mind: Clearing Away Mental Dust

Let's say that Anne has had a series of unsuccessful romantic relationships that all follow the same pattern: each relationship ends with the other person telling her she's too challenging, defensive, moody, or angry. Though she recognizes that they are referring to specific incidents—for she does have her fair share of bad moods—she doesn't understand why all her relationships end, and in such an antagonizing way. Why me? she asks. And her circular life continues.

There are times in life when we see everything clearly. Things just fall into place in our minds, and we know exactly how we must move forward with something. But how often do we have those moments? Maybe once every couple of years? If the mind is in the way, we have to rely on these moments coming up involuntarily—which usually doesn't happen when we're distraught and hurt over a breakup. With self-study, we can create such moments.

The first step in self-study within the realm of the mind is to get to know who you are. Or, perhaps more accurately, observe what your mind attaches to in any given moment. When we experience a situation, we have thoughts about that situation. The texture of these thoughts is as varied as we are—it's the nature of our thoughts that defines our personality.

For example, three different people could all be waiting for a city bus at the bus stop. One person might have anxious, fearful thoughts about what will happen if they're late, another person might have grateful thoughts about how they have time to spend reading their novel before they get to work, and yet another person could be really mad that the bus is a whole minute late and intensely angry about the city's general incompetence. But depending on the nature of the situation and the nature of the person in that situation, these thoughts could be unwanted, like the angry and anxious thoughts, or completely welcome, like the grateful thoughts.

Self-study instructs us to simply observe our thoughts and become aware of them. You might feel anger in response to a situation, but that anger goes away when the situation goes away. Those angry thoughts are not you; your ego created them when it felt it had lost control. When you become aware of your thoughts and recognize that they aren't you, you are able to observe them as workings of the mind. In doing this, you become aware of the thought, and just as you might replace the potato chips and cookies in your diet with carrots and cauliflower, you replace these thoughts with something that is opposite in quality. You let go of the angry thought and think of something that induces calm.

We often repeat patterns in our lives, just like Anne did. Without practicing self-study, the ego tells us a story and we feel hurt, betrayed, or annoyed when someone says something about who he or she thinks we are. We might feel anxious about a late bus, or just indifferent. We might feel enticed by fast food advertisements, or repulsed. But when we simply embrace the fact that our thoughts are not us, we can observe the thoughts our ego is creating, much like we might watch a leaf float by on a small river or stream. When we watch these thoughts pass us by, we learn from the experience.

Let's say you just went through a breakup and, like Anne's situation, your ex-partner said something hurtful about your anger and intensity. You might experience an initial moment of pain, but after you recognize that your thoughts are separate from you, you can see from a more detached place that your ex isn't being mean or hurtful but is simply experiencing his own pain and has entered your life to help you learn something about yourself. A moment, a month, or a year later, a new awareness might emerge regarding the patterns you've been perpetuating throughout your life. Instead of the same hurtful things happening again, you learn that you're repeatedly attracting a certain type of person into your life to teach you how you might emerge from your personal suffering. As you let go of the need to analyze, deduce, or intellectualize why certain things keep happening, you start to discover the truth of your own existence. You no longer ask, "Why me?" Instead you create space to observe what's happening to you and allow yourself to see everything clearly. You remove each layer of dust covering who you are and reveal the clear glass underneath.

The Spirit: Revealing the Glass Underneath

Each of us is a reflection of the Creative Spirit. We each have divine perfection within us. Jesus asked how you can presume to help another see clearly by removing the speck in that person's eye when you have an entire log in your own eye. By observing our bodies and our minds, we begin to clear the dust, specks, or logs away. We recognize that intuition comes from being guided by the Spirit.

Over time, our observations will lead to truth, and we will have an intuitive knowledge of how to live as a reflection of that truth. When we observe ourselves, we stop identifying ourselves as the mind and intuitively grasp that the Spirit is everything. We start to see the mind, body, and senses for what they are—a transitory experience—and we detach from these things as not being lasting or real. When we finally see clearly, we are able to help others clear their eyes of everything that obstructs what they see.

The Plan

To begin your practice of self-study, you will train yourself to observe your body and then your mind. In observing without forcing an analytical deduction, you allow an intuitive awareness of your body and mind to emerge. One day you have no clear sense of what you must do to continue on your path, then the next day something emerges from within. You begin to know your true nature.

The Realm of the Body

Observing the body is far more straightforward than observing the mind. When we observe our skin being dry, it doesn't take a tremendously involved intuitive process to determine that the body needs moisturizing. In this step, you can seek guidance and feedback from a trained Ayurvedic practitioner or learn to be patient and allow information to emerge through your intuition.

You will benefit from self-study of the body if you do not know what your prakruti is, if you have no idea what imbalances you have in your body, or if you've never considered the source of your day-to-day discomforts beyond what your doctor has told you.

The outside of the body is a map to what is happening inside. Everything from the eyes to the tongue tells us which elements are out of balance, what sort of toxicity has built up, and what our prakruti is. To begin this process, determine your prakruti by answering the following questions. Keep track of your answers on a piece of paper.

1. My bodily proportions are
   a. thin and lanky.
   b. medium-sized and symmetrical.
   c. large and stocky.

2. My joints
   a. are weak and tend to crack.
   b. are loose.
   c. are large and tend to be padded.

3. In food, I am drawn to
    a. sweet, sour, and salty tastes.
    b. sweet, bitter, and astringent tastes.
    c. pungent, bitter, and astringent tastes.

4. I describe my skin as
    a. dry and rough.
    b. soft and warm.
    c. oily and moist.

5. I describe my hair as
    a. dry and brittle.
    b. fine and thin.
    c. thick and abundant.

6. I describe my fingernails as
    a. brittle and cracked.
    b. pink and soft.
    c. wide and thick.

7. I describe my eyes as
    a. small and dry.
    b. reddish and sensitive.
    c. white and wide open.

8. I describe my appetite as
    a. changing depending on how I'm feeling.
    b. strong and excessive.
    c. low but consistent.

9. I describe my digestion as
    a. very delicate and disturbed by many foods.
    b. efficient and accommodating of many different foods.
    c. slow.

10. I describe my stool as
    a. small and hard.
    b. loose and sometimes burning.
    c. solid and heavy.

11. The environment that tends to cause me the greatest discomfort is
    a. a cold day.

b. a hot day.

c. a wet and humid day.

Tally up the number of a's, b's, and c's you marked. If you have the greatest number of a's, then you likely have a predominantly Vata constitution. If you have the greatest number of b's, you have a predominantly Pitta constitution. If you have the greatest number of c's, you have a predominantly Kapha constitution. In addition to this quiz, there are other ways to determine your prakruti.

THE PULSE. The pulse is a key diagnostic tool for Ayurvedic practitioners. When they check a patient's pulse, they're able to determine not only aspects of the patient's prakruti but also their general state of health. This technique takes years to master. However, you may gain some insight into your own body if you take your own pulse. Press the pointer, middle, and index fingers of one hand onto the pulse of the opposite wrist to feel the pulse's beat. Is it subtle, erratic, fast, and snake-like like a Vata pulse? Is it decisive, strong, consistent, and frog-like like a Pitta pulse? Is it slow, calm, flowing, and swan-like like a Kapha pulse?

THE SKIN. The skin and other parts of the body indicate not just your basic nature but the current state of your health. Are there any outbreaks or other problematic symptoms? This means you have imbalanced digestion. Is your skin dry and prone to causing pain? These are Vata qualities. Is it prone to irritation, and does it feel very warm? These are Pitta qualities. Does your skin feel oily and itchy? These are Kapha qualities.

THE EYES. Your eyes can be a source of information about your current state as well. Are your eyes dry, or do they seem to water a lot? This means they have a Vata issue. Are they burning and prone to redness? This means they have a Pitta issue. Are they itchy or have a film over them? This means they have a Kapha issue.

THE TONGUE. The tongue indicates exactly where toxicity is located in the body and can provide extensive information. A clean, pink tongue indicates that the system isn't overburdened with toxicity; a tongue with a darkish coating indicates a Vata imbalance; a tongue with a greenish or yellowish coating indicates a Pitta imbalance; a tongue with a whitish coating indicates a Kapha imbalance. A coating concentrated in the back of the tongue indicates toxicity in the large intestine, while a coating in the middle of the tongue indicates toxicity in the stomach or small intestine. A coating toward the front of the tongue is related to toxicity in the lungs and heart.

Your task for these two weeks is quite simple: each morning, after you've practiced your morning purity routine, you are to take inventory of what you observe about these various aspects of your body. On the first day, take the quiz and listen to your pulse. What would you say your prakruti is? Then, each day, take note of your skin, eyes, and tongue. What does this information suggest to you? Do you feel any pain or discomfort inside? Are you suffering from any chronic ailments or sources of discomfort?

Without the guidance of an Ayurvedic practitioner, it will likely take a long time to begin shifting your body into a more balanced state. What is most important is to observe your body for these two weeks and beyond. As you take in this information on a regular basis, you will begin to intuitively grasp what needs to be done next.

The Realm of the Mind

As you might imagine, training yourself to observe your mind is difficult. You may find yourself saying something like, "Okay, I observed my thoughts to be angry, and I don't like them. Now what?" It's this last part, the "now what?" that will be a challenge to let go of. You may find through observation that your thoughts lead to annoyance, but the way to create change—pursuing something that is the opposite of what is already there—will reveal itself intuitively. During these two weeks, you will begin a self-study of the mind using two methods: 1) you will observe your thoughts as you encounter emotionally noteworthy situations, and 2) you will read spiritual material.

OBSERVING THOUGHTS

When we encounter emotionally significant situations, our thoughts often go all over the place. If we're late for something, we start to worry about our tardiness. If we get good news, we become excited and jubilant. During these two weeks, train yourself to observe your thoughts whenever you encounter emotionally significant situations. Emotionally significant situations you might encounter include the following:

- You are woken up in the middle of the night by loud neighbors.

- You win a large sum of money in an office pool.

- You are late for work.

- You get a bonus at work.

- You get knocked around in a crowded bus or train during rush hour.

- You meet someone you find attractive.

- You get a parking ticket.

- Your child wins recognition at school.

- You lose your wallet.

- Someone finds your wallet.

- You sprain your ankle.

- You get promoted.

- Your limo is late.

- Someone insults you.

- You sell a manuscript or another project to someone.

- You get in a car accident.

- You lose your job.

- You fall in love.

- A loved one gets hurt.

- A loved one survives a dangerous situation.

Without self-study, your ego will step in when you experience one of these situations—whether it is bad, like losing your wallet, or good, like finding it. Either way, when you allow the emotions that surround such a situation to dominate your thoughts, you're really just allowing your mind to step up and try to control the situation. And since your ego won't ever be able to control the outside world, you won't ever be at peace. Use the Presence Practice each morning to focus on the idea that your thoughts are not you, and therefore you can let them come up and simply watch them float down the river. Questions you may ask yourself when doing the Presence Practice include these:

- What sorts of situations get me most upset?

- What sorts of situations make me most jubilant and cheerful?

- When I get upset, am I more prone to anger, sadness, worry, grief, fear, anxiety, or something else?

- When I am cheerful, am I more prone to excitement, mania, self-aggrandizement, self-righteousness, or something else?

Consider focusing one day on situations that make you upset and the next day on those that make you cheerful. Either way, you're allowing your mind to be swept away by your emotions, but when you observe your thoughts in emotional situations—and the reactions that ensue—you will become aware of how you might fill your mind instead with more peaceful, balanced thoughts. From here, you will begin to intuit ways to find this peace in your life and yourself.

READING SPIRITUAL MATERIAL

The Sanskrit term *svadhyaya* may be understood to mean reading spiritual material as a way to remove the dust from the glass. This can be any material that has been conceived through self-realization, such as the Yoga Sutras, the Bhagavad Gita, or the Vedas, or material like the Jatakas, the Torah, the I Ching, Christ's words, Buddhist teachings, or the Qur'an.

Here in the West, people read to take in information or for entertainment. We read something, and then we're done with it. But reading the Gita and other spiritual material requires us to reread it again and again so that we may remove the layers of dust and uncover its truth from within. Thus it is also a practice of observation. Just like we observe thoughts in response to a stressful situation instead of attaching to them, we observe the words of spiritual material and, rather than attaching to an idea of understanding it right away, we allow the Spirit to work in its own time as we intuit its true meaning.

In addition to spending a few minutes each day reminding yourself to observe your thoughts, your task for these two weeks is to spend five minutes at the end of each night reading the Gita, the Yoga Sutras, the Vedas, or another spiritual text. Simply read the material for five minutes before going to bed, and let go of any need to understand it. Though I suggest only five minutes, you can add as much time as you like. As you continue this practice over time, you will not simply understand it but experience it.

The Realm of the Spirit

The work of self-study in the realm of the spirit begins when you experience your body to be nothing more than a vessel for your divine light, when your mind is nothing more than a transitory distraction that behaves like a five-year-old demanding your attention while you're on the phone. Here the glass tabletop is nearly clear. You see a computer, a car, the sages, the Gita, yourself, and everything else as consciousness. Everything comes from the Spirit.

After you have sustained a practice of observing and reading spiritual material for several years, you will take steps to embody the realm of the spirit. Your practice is to place yourself in the middle of the busiest, noisiest, most chaotic situations you can find and stay there for years. You might even move to a specific place in which you will be useful in your work even though it is chaotic to a mind that isn't controlled. Similar to how a Yogi like His Holiness the Dalai Lama lives in the circular world but conducts his work by traveling across the globe, you will be able to live and exist anywhere and live out of spirit. You will know when it is time for you to begin your work on this realm, for it will come to you naturally. You will begin to see those who would otherwise overwhelm you as also being the Spirit. You will see them all as the same as yourself.

With clear glass, you don't impose your own layer of dust on anything. You continue to watch your thoughts, and you continue to read spiritual material. And no matter what you do in any given moment, your study of yourself always reveals you to be a perfect source of light.

Emerging as a Masterpiece

After the intensity of austerity practices, the addition of self-study will be relatively simple and accessible. Because you've pursued this program for several months now, it will likely feel less like a specific part of your day and more like a lifestyle. Your work in observing yourself may be difficult, but with the support of the habits you've been forming, you are likely to become more aware of yourself and your actions than you ever were before. As you continue with your self-study, you will become more and more open to the Spirit guiding you.

Putting It Together

If you are practicing exclusively in the realm of the body, your practice over these two weeks will look like this:

- Observe the state of your body and its various features. If you are so inclined, seek out an Ayurvedic practitioner to help you find out more about the nature of your dosha type and your body as a whole.

- Continue your daily purity practices each morning.

- Take herbal tea twice a day to continue building strength and cleanliness.

And remember . . .

- Continue eating half as much processed food and unhealthy substances as you did prior to the program, avoid eating during the last two hours of the day, and release your sexual essence half as often as you did before Week 7. Continue to avoid accumulating possessions.

- Continue building your nonviolence, truthfulness, and nonstealing behaviors to the best of your ability. Continue participating in a physical activity that requires presence of mind at least once every two weeks.

- Eat your lunch in silence at least once a week. Go for a brief walk or jog as well.

- Consider fasting for a day during these two weeks.

If you are practicing exclusively within the realm of the mind, your daily practice over these two weeks will look like this:

- Spend ten minutes of your morning repeating the Gayatri Mantra.

- Continue to accept insulting situations as an opportunity to burn off mental toxins, but now use your Presence Practice to remind yourself to observe your thoughts in response to emotional situations.

- Read the Yoga Sutras or other spiritual material for five minutes before you go to bed.

And remember . . .

- Continue eating natural foods, refrain from eating in the last five hours of the day and after 7 P.M., and continue to have sex in moderation.

- Continue your nonviolence, truthfulness, and nonstealing practices, and avoid sexual thoughts. Continue to let go of attachments to people and situations that you are keeping out of fear.

- Continue to take note of your situational desires, and create alternate possibilities for your life in response.

- Consider fasting for one day each week.

the higher purpose

SELF-SURRENDER

AFGHANISTAN IS NOT A BUILT-UP PLACE. IN KABUL, ITS CAPITAL AND largest city, you'll find a number of large, beautiful mosques, but otherwise there are few signs of development. Tanks and blockades are everywhere. You'll see concrete walls. You'll see Camp Phoenix, Kabul Military Training Center, and other military installations. But it's the unexpected things that can really make you take notice of your situation.

In 2011, I traveled to Afghanistan to introduce soldiers, students, and street children to the Yogic path. With so many years of violence tainting the country's recent past and the prospect of international soldiers pulling out of the country in a few years, it seemed more important than ever that Afghans have as many tools as possible for living in peace. They were responsive to the teachings. Some of the soldiers I taught worked at prisons holding dangerous terrorists, and they commented that Yoga postures and meditation would help the prisoners overcome their hate.

Toward the end of my time there, my companion, Amandine, made arrangements for me to teach a man who had been one of the most ferocious fighters of the Taliban regime. As an international peacekeeper, Amandine had met him before and was able to make an appointment. We were instructed via phone to take a taxi to a specified location about a half hour outside of Kabul, at which point we would receive further instructions.

The taxi let us out in an area with a number of apartment buildings, and we had to call a different phone number to be told where to go. This was a precaution to prevent members of terrorist organizations from tapping phone conversations. There was much fear of spies—especially with unknown visitors like us. We finally reached the building we were instructed to go to, climbed the stairs, and knocked on the door. A lady greeted us at the door, and we were taken to a back room and told to have a seat on the carpet and wait.

Eventually, a middle-aged man with a full, grizzly beard came into the room. His face showed he had known war his entire life. He greeted us in Pashtun, one of Afghanistan's main languages. I grew up in Iran, and my knowledge of Farsi enabled me to speak to most people around Kabul in their language of Dari. But we had brought a translator to speak to this man. We all sat down, and I explained why we were there and what we hoped to achieve. As I spoke, he glared at me. He then spoke, and the translator followed: "To turn destruction into construction, into peace and upward mobility. That is his mission." This man may have been known as a ferocious commander, but he had now laid down his arms. I recounted my sense of how we can attain peace and commented on how peaceful so many Afghans already are. "We have to work for it," the man responded. "To achieve peace, you have to mobilize the society. It's not easy, but it's attainable."

We continued to speak about how it might be possible to overcome the many obstacles that are part of a peace-building process. As the translator explained something that the man said, a young girl came in to cuddle with him and shyly glanced at us. He gave her an affectionate pat as she whispered something to him. When he heard the translator relay the last thing I had said, he smiled. "We must use our intellect," he said, "not guns. We've lost our loved ones again and again. I don't want our Afghan sisters and brothers to lose their loved ones either. Now it's time for us to stop this."

This man had rejected his life of destruction because he no longer wanted to create a violent world for his granddaughter—the young girl who had come in to visit us. I took a few minutes to explain how to concentrate on the breath as a first step toward meditation, and we sat together in silence for a while. Even after Amandine and I had finished and were ready to resume the conversation, he kept his eyes closed for some time longer.

In Afghanistan, you'll see many things. You'll see tanks and concrete barricades, mosques and food markets. After getting dropped off by a taxi in a strange place, using a phone line that we hoped was not tapped, and putting myself in a situation that could very well have been dangerous, I found a man who demonstrated that change is possible. Since I had no fear, I had an opportunity to hear what an ex-Taliban commander thought about his first experience with meditation. "It was delightful," he said.

The Forfeit of Control

I could have told you a very different story with the same events. I could have told you a harrowing tale of holding my breath as I passed intimidating military complexes, looking around to see if we were being tracked as we got out of the cab, and almost running from the most ferocious man I'd ever seen. I could have told a story that showed me crippled with fear and digging deep inside myself to surmount that fear and become the heroic savior of the day.

And why not tell this story? Shouldn't a trip to an ex-Taliban commander's home be filled with trepidation and imminent danger? After all, Afghanistan has been one of the most volatile and unpredictable parts of the world for decades. My time there was no exception: a suicide bomber jumped in front of Amandine's 4x4 when she went to pick me up at the airport. This is a daily occurrence in Afghanistan.

Through the practices we've explored in this program, we've seen how the ego incites emotional reactions to situations. Whether it's the anger felt in response to violence, the apprehension felt in the face of a lack of truthfulness, the desire felt after discontentment, or any number of other harmful emotions, the ego coerces us into thinking that we must try to control situations we are in or we won't be happy. And yet any one of those emotions leads to suffering and unhappiness.

Let's say that two people are in a car driving through Kabul, and a suicide bomber runs in front of the vehicle. The first person feels intense anxiety and fear, but the other person experiences peace and contentment. Both people have experienced the same threat to their safety, and yet their reactions are different. Though the suicide bomber fails in his task and neither person's safety is ultimately compromised, one person has suffered and one person has felt only peace. Were these two people to continue to respond to life in the same way they did in that moment, one would continue to experience anxious thoughts ("What if I'm hurt? What if I die?"), and the other would continue to use each moment to experience peace. If they lived for the same amount of time, what would be the primary difference between their lives? Only their perception of the time they have here on earth.

Whenever we succumb to fear, we are succumbing to the power of our own egos. This is what would have happened if I had approached the ex-Taliban commander's home with fear and trepidation: "What if this is just a trap to kidnap a westerner, and what if I'm hurt or killed? My life is too important for me to die now." This trepidation would represent my ego telling me that I needed to control the outcome of my endeavor in order for it to be successful, because if I were harmed in any way, then my ego would lose control and I would experience significant pain.

When we set out on an endeavor because of what we feel we can get out of it, whether it's the money we get from a job, the pleasure we get from entertainment, or the recognition we get from charitable acts, we set ourselves up for a painful roller coaster of emotions. We might feel slighted when we don't get as much money as we feel we're worth, we might feel disappointed by a night out that was supposed to be fabulous, or we might feel underappreciated by those we seek to help. We experience these emotions because pursuing an endeavor out of desire for its promised benefits comes from our ego trying to control the world around us and enforce rule over the spirit. Had I gone to Afghanistan and then to the commander's house with a desire to feel valuable for having committed myself to a meaningful act, then I would have been acting to gratify my ego. My ego would have needed to be in control, and a suicide attack would have robbed my ego of that control. In response to this false sense of control, my ego would have compelled me to feel fear, anxiety, or some other product of my mind until its control was no longer threatened.

Instead, I felt peace. I was able to observe the potential threat to my safety, but I didn't feel any particular emotion in response. I just pursued the task in front of me, whether it was climbing stairs or speaking with the grizzled man. I remained present to the moment, and in doing so I was able to replace fear with action. I was able to do this through an act of surrender to the Creative Spirit.

The final practice of Patanjali's observations is self-surrender, or *ishvarapranidhana*. In the previous two weeks, we explored observing and letting go of harmful emotions; self-surrender calls on us to accept everything that happens in our lives as part of the greater plan of the perfection of the Creative Spirit. As the creative force behind all of existence, this presence—whether we call it nature, energy, God, or something else—is a perfect entity. It created water, fire, flowers, birds, and everything else in the natural world to be exactly what they needed to be. Since we are born, live, and die as an extension of this force, everything that happens to this body and mind is likewise part of the Creative Spirit. Therefore, everything we experience in life is divine and can serve us as we find our way to self-realization. When we embrace our bodies and minds as containers for the part of us that is as perfect as everything else in nature, we can focus our intentions surrounding any given task or endeavor to be in reverence for this force. Whether we live a short time or a long time, with a strong body or a disabled one, everything that happens to us is godly and has a purpose.

Now, that might be a lovely, high-minded ideal for people in India wearing orange robes, but what does it mean in our modern lives of working through lunch, remembering doctor appointments, and shopping for groceries? If everything that happens in life is part of the greater plan of divine perfection, then to practice self-surrender is to do these things as well as everything else in service to that plan. Rather than seeking out a job for the money we will get from it, we seek it as an opportunity to serve those who will benefit from our services. Rather than looking at family members and friends as people who can provide us with joy or fulfillment, we look at them as someone to serve. Rather than committing to a charitable act because of the recognition we will receive, we do so in an effort to selflessly serve another person.

How did I feel peace that day in Afghanistan? By accepting that whatever happened to me that day, it was all part of an already perfect plan. That my life has been part of this perfection since it began.

Closing the Gap

The idea of surrendering everything in life to a higher purpose may sound inspiring and uplifting in theory, but here in the modern world it's often difficult to let go of the cynicism that so many of us feel when we hear such things. The work we do on this path is often defined by a seemingly enormous gap between where we are in our lives at this moment and where we might be after a lifetime of pursuing these practices. How can we let go of traumatic experiences, like Somaly Mam did in her nonviolence practice, or commit an act of nonstealing, like the bishop in *Les Misérables*? How can we learn to do everything in life in service to a higher force—and to all humanity as an extension of that higher force? Fortunately, the first steps in a practice of self-surrender will meet us where we are in the realm of the body. As with the other abstentions and observations, the practice grows from there.

The Body: Contained Self-Surrender

If the ultimate goal of self-surrender is for everything we do to be of service to a higher purpose, we get started on this path in the realm of the body by physically placing ourselves in situations intended as an exercise in service. In other words, we take a small step toward the larger goal of total surrender by committing a finite period of time to service toward another. We might spend a couple of hours of our Saturday volunteering and then allow ourselves to enjoy a movie afterward. We might usually come home after a long day of work and just plop ourselves in front of Facebook, but now we first spend an hour attending to family members before chatting with friends.

If we limit our service to specific tasks, committing ourselves to these ideals won't seem so daunting. But then, when the ego shows up—as it inevitably will—we tap into our self-study practice from Weeks 17–18: "I came here to volunteer at this soup kitchen to help others, and that man I just served gave me the nastiest look. Doesn't he know that I could be off shopping or hanging out with my friends right now, instead of serving him food? What nerve he has to— Oh, wait. That's my ego. I'm here to serve another person, and that man seems like he could really use some support. Let us continue."

The Mind: Uncontained Self-Surrender

Whereas in the realm of the body there may be a physical separation between an act of service and the rest of life ("Now I'm going to go volunteer"), there is no separation in the realm of the mind. In the mental realm, we are training our minds to embrace everything we do as an opportunity to be of service to others.

This means that your role among the people you encounter in your personal and professional lives is to serve them. You might still volunteer for charitable works, but that activity isn't any different from making a meal at home for your family, which you prepare conscientiously and with their benefit in mind. Your job, though it may earn you money, is no less valid if you earn less or no money at all. Whether you are a plumber or a writer, you offer your services to all people whether they can pay you or not (though what's funny is that those who commit themselves to this level of service wind up attracting more clients and creating greater material abundance in their lives). If you work for a company that is doing a disservice to the world, perhaps through ecologically destructive manufacturing practices or abusive policies toward employees and competitors, you find another company in which to offer your skills.

When you are frustrated, angry, sad, or disappointed, you remind yourself that the work isn't for you but for humanity and for the Creative Spirit to express itself. You don't ever give at your own expense (depriving yourself of sleep, food, health, or your personal practice), but all your conduct beyond personal preservation is a commitment to others. Your self-preservation is a service to the Spirit as well. In the realm of the mind, you ask a simple question of everything you do: is this good for everybody? If it's not, you switch it out for an endeavor that is.

The Spirit: On a Spinning Wheel

I would like you to take a moment to consider Mohandas Gandhi. If you're like most people, when you think of Gandhi you probably think of peaceful resistance, Indian liberation, nonviolence, and wisdom, or maybe you just think of the actor Ben Kingsley. Most people associate Gandhi with these things because his time on earth epitomized the life of self-surrender. When he saw the oppressive nature of British rule over the Indian subcontinent, Gandhi committed his life to liberating the country and doing so in a peaceful way. Everything he did was in service to his country. When he learned of people taking up arms and perpetrating violent conflicts, he fasted until the violence stopped. He spent hours on a spinning wheel making his own clothes, as this action represented the self-sufficiency he hoped for his country to attain.

When we practice self-surrender in the realm of the body, we set aside time to serve others. In the realm of the mind, we do whatever it is we do but with the intention to serve others. Self-surrender in the highest realm, however, requires that we form our life's work around service to the rest of the world. We no longer own a home or any other earthly possessions that serve our own well-being. Instead we possess only that which enables us to serve others. Here, we let go of control and move from the head into the heart. Whether we commit ourselves to peaceful protest or teach people in developing nations how to grow their own food, everything we do is in recognition that the Creative Spirit has a plan for us and all we can do is follow its perfect lead.

The Plan

Self-surrender is an ambitious practice to incorporate into one's life. The ego runs strong: it doesn't want to lose control, and it doesn't want to give in to the Spirit. However, the practices you've done in the first eighteen weeks of this program have helped you center yourself, making you available for this level of service. You will chip away at the body and eventually the mind; you will then experience the peace that comes from letting go of the ego and embracing total devotion to the Creative Spirit.

The Realm of the Body

Your task for these two weeks is relatively simple to describe but ambitious in scope. Once a day for the next two weeks, you are to commit to one task of service to another person in your life. This may be a family member, such as your spouse or child, or it may be a coworker, the beneficiary of a charity you volunteer for, or even a total stranger. Your work is to carry out this task, observing your feelings as you do so. If intense emotions come up during or after this work, allow them to happen and then let them go. Possible ways to serve others during these two weeks include the following:

- Spend an hour playing a game with your children or helping them complete a task important to them.

- Spend an hour providing your spouse with assistance in completing some task.

- Prepare a meal for your family that would usually be reserved for a special occasion.

- Take on a chore typically managed by another family member.

- Volunteer at a soup kitchen.

- Volunteer at an assisted living home.

- Volunteer at a homeless or transitional shelter.

- Volunteer at a hospital.

- Donate your time at a nonprofit organization that doesn't have a specifically charitable mission (theater, school, museum, community development center).

- Offer professional services to a nonprofit organization.

- Offer professional services to a client free of charge.

- Commit a random act of kindness toward another person you encounter as you go through your day—especially if you're not very fond of them.

These two weeks will give you a taste of practicing self-surrender on a small scale. I recommend that you sustain this practice by committing to at least a couple of hours of service each week moving forward. You will benefit most from moving on to the realm of the mind when you're able to consistently let go of your thoughts during acts of service for months at a time. When you no longer feel attached to people seeming grateful, to getting credit for your work, or to other thoughts that come from the ego, you're ready to move along to the realm of the mind.

The Realm of the Mind

Self-surrender practice in the realm of the mind begins with the intention that everything you do be in service to others. At the end of this process, you will have committed all actions to the Creative Spirit. Since there is a great disparity between these points, self-surrender is a sizable task that will likely take years to develop. Therefore, your work during these two weeks is to take a first step. Self-surrender may be applied to various aspects of your life. During these two weeks, experiment with the following areas of your life:

PROFESSIONAL: I work on a sliding scale based on the amount of money the client has. In doing this work not for money but to help the client, I'm serving. But as soon as I start basing my availability not on how I can serve another person but on how much money I can get, I fall back into living to fulfill my own ego. You too can shift your intentions to reflect this practice. If you work freelance, replace a set fee schedule with a fee based on the client's means. If you are employed by others, commit yourself to working only for a company that satisfactorily considers ecological preservation and provides goods or services that are healthy and of genuine service to humanity. If you are not currently working for such a company, start researching new job opportunities.

RECREATIONAL: Let go of any hobbies pursued for personal gratification and instead conduct all activities for the benefit of others (for instance, if you make things, donate some of them to a group that can fund-raise with them).

CHARITABLE: Commit yourself to daily selfless acts for the benefit of others in lieu of personal entertainment.

NUTRITIONAL: Let go of eating for pleasure and sense gratification, and eat food only for its nourishment and medicinal qualities. Eat only vegetarian food so as to utilize fewer resources (water, grain, life, etc.).

PHYSICAL: Let go of any exercise or other physical regimen that doesn't serve your personal practice (such as rigorous exercises designed to shape and tone the body). Avoid looking in the mirror except to shave or quickly groom yourself.

CREATIVE: If you are creatively inclined, give your creations to others without trying to make money or receive recognition. Consider distributing them anonymously and donating the proceeds to a charitable organization.

INTERPERSONAL: Commit yourself to every relationship as an exercise in complete service. This is perhaps the most complex practice, for the entire process is based on giving. Commit all time not used for work and self-preservation (including personal practice) for the benefit of your family, friends, and neighbors.

ENVIRONMENTAL: Work with nature in mind. If your work, your workplace, or the products you make are polluting the earth, take steps to change your work and do what must be done to benefit the earth.

Any one of these tasks requires significant effort to shift away from the need for ego gratification. Spend these two weeks experimenting with as many or as few of them as you like, but by the end of the two weeks commit to one and move forward accordingly.

To help you in this endeavor, use your morning Presence Practice to detach from the emotions that will inevitably accompany many of these tasks. As you sit quietly each morning, ask yourself the following questions:

- When someone doesn't seem to appreciate my work, is it more important for me to get that recognition or to simply enjoy doing the work?

- In trying new endeavors, do I have expectations for what those endeavors will do for me, or am I able to let go of such attachments?

- What compels me to pursue a change in this area of my life?

- What sort of reactions have I had to pursuing such endeavors in the past? Disappointment? Frustration? Pride?

In exploring endeavors for a higher purpose, you will learn to let go of adverse emotional reactions you encounter along the way.

The Realm of the Spirit

If you looked at two cups filled with tea, you would see them as separate. One cup could be served to one person, and the other cup could be served to another. What would happen, though, if you combined them into one larger cup? Would you still see them as separate? You would not. You would see them as one. When you practice self-surrender in the realm of the spirit, you see everything as an extension of that spirit. Everything from a beautiful flower to a diaper filled with poo is energy and light—everything goes together like one cup of tea. Even man-made things were at one point minerals and other resources provided by the earth that we took and made into things. This is where we take ourselves when we practice self-surrender in the highest realm. An alchemist turns the most basic elements into gold, for he knows that all elements are aspects of the Creative Spirit. When you practice self-surrender in this realm, you become a spiritual alchemist: nothing can be separated from light.

To experience self-surrender in this realm, your work is to begin seeing all things as divine. When you are able to see a flower, your iPhone, or even a pile of poo as part of the same spirit, you are on your way to accepting everything that happens to you and everyone else as part of the master plan. Whether you live in the smallest cave or the largest city, everything you do is in service to a higher force that may then help others alleviate their suffering. You donate not just 5 percent of your earnings but all your earnings. You stop doing anything that isn't good for the earth. You have no emotional reaction to your life ending now or in thirty years, for everything that happens is part of the same spirit.

Emerging as a Masterpiece

As the final aspect of the abstentions and observations, your practice of self-surrender rounds out a particularly ambitious practice that will ultimately lead you to experience greater joy in your life. Ask yourself how you are doing with this work. Do you feel an inclination to rush through these practices in favor of the ones that are yet to come? Are you struggling to see how they fit into your life as a whole? Do you wish the One Plan didn't challenge you so much? Commitment to the practices in these first twenty weeks of this plan will change your view of life completely, so remember that this is groundwork for your whole life. With devotion to the practice of self-surrender, you will begin to experience life not as a source of anxiety and fear, but as a source of peace.

Putting It Together

If you are practicing exclusively in the realm of the body, these two weeks will look like this:

- Continue your daily purity practices each morning. Observe the state of your skin, tongue, and other features.

- Take herbal tea twice a day to continue building strength and cleanliness.

- Commit some time each day to an act of service toward a family member, friend, colleague, or someone else who crosses your path.

And remember . . .

- Continue eating half as much processed food and unhealthy substances as you did prior to the program. Avoid eating during the last two hours of the day, and release your sexual essence half as often as you did before Week 7. Continue to avoid accumulating possessions, and observe the state of your body.

- Continue building your nonviolence, truthfulness, and nonstealing behaviors to the best of your ability. Continue participating in a physical activity that requires presence of mind at least once every two weeks.

- Eat your lunch in silence at least once a week. Go for a brief walk or jog.

- Consider fasting for a day during these two weeks.

If you are practicing exclusively in the realm of the mind, your daily practice over these two weeks will look like this:

- Spend ten minutes of your morning repeating the Gayatri Mantra.

- Choose one area of your life in which to commit to a practice of self-surrender.

- Read the Yoga Sutras or other spiritual material for five minutes before you go to bed.

And remember . . .

- Continue eating natural foods, refrain from eating during the last five hours of the day and after 7 P.M., and continue to have sex in moderation.

- Continue your nonviolence, truthfulness, and nonstealing practices, and avoid sexual thoughts. Continue to let go of attachments to people and situations that you are keeping out of fear, and observe your thoughts.

- Continue to take note of your situational desires and create alternate possibilities for your life, and continue to observe your thoughts in emotionally heightened situations.

- Consider fasting for one day each week.

building on the path

TAKE A MOMENT TO PICTURE YOURSELF BEFORE YOU BEGAN WEEK 1 of this program. What were you eating? What were your thoughts about other people? These first twenty weeks of the program may not have been filled with hours of physical exercises, but they more than likely offered you a new way to look at the world around you and the role you play in it. It has also mentally prepared you for the next phase of the plan. Very few people ever notice or do very much about the fact that they have a life worth exploring on a deeper level. Having gone through this transformation means that you are now one of the few. Congratulations.

The remaining thirty-two weeks of this program are devoted to practices more commercially known as Yoga, such as postures and breathing. Whereas much of the work in the first twenty weeks of the One Plan is oriented toward altering behaviors, shifting attitudes, and other nuanced actions, most of the work you will do in the remainder of the program is based on crafting a regimen that will play a more active, outward role in your lifestyle. You will gradually add exercises and techniques, and in cultivating these practices you'll enhance your capacity for living in health, balance, and joy.

We will cover six more branches of Patanjali's Eightfold Path in the remaining thirty-two weeks, divided into four sections of eight weeks each. Even though you've already spent nearly five months grounding yourself in beneficial behaviors, it can still be difficult to make such a sizable commitment. For this reason, these practices have been spaced out over more than half the year to give you an opportunity to build this routine gradually.

The practices outlined in part 4 are divided into the realms of the body, mind, and spirit, so you will be able to pursue each practice in a way that is appropriate and beneficial for wherever you're at in your life. You may already have an established posture practice but haven't practiced sense control. You will then benefit from practicing postures in the realm of the mind but sense control in the realm of the body. No matter how you choose to pursue these practices, though, part 4 has been organized to ensure that you have a fruitful and consistent experience for the remainder of your time exploring and practicing the One Plan.

unifying a divided house

POSTURES

When you hear the word *YOGA*, what is the first thing you think of? Do you think of a self-realized sage who laid out aphoristic strands of truth about ancient traditions? Do you think of nonviolence, purity, or self-surrender? No, what you probably envision is a sleek-looking studio with new age music playing and people stretching themselves into very beautiful but highly unlikely positions and shapes. What you probably think of is Yoga postures.

There are many people in the West—myself included—who were introduced to Yoga through physical postures. We see people stretch and strengthen their bodies in Yoga studios, gyms, workshops, or retreats. As of this writing, there are some fifteen million people who practice Yoga in America alone. That's a lot of strengthening and stretching. But most of the people going to studios are practicing postures before committing to nonviolence, contentment, and the rest of the abstentions and observations. They may be going to studios, but they're doing little else from the Yogic path.

The One Plan provides a way for you to follow the path that Patanjali set out over two thousand years ago. This program reflects modern life without omitting any traditions. What typically happens with spiritual messages is that the messenger—be it Moses, the Buddha, or Jesus Christ—describes a path toward self-realization, but the message is reinterpreted in various ways by people who suffered on account of their ego and altered the teachings based on their limited understanding of or commitment to the practices. Christ advised his followers that "if a house is divided against itself, that house cannot stand" (Mark 3:25), and yet there are nearly forty thousand denominations of Christianity in the world. Like Moses, the Buddha, and Jesus Christ, Patanjali set out to share his message through a process of self-realization that has been reinterpreted in different ways. When modern Western culture embraced Yoga in the twentieth century, we reduced Patanjali's system to the physical side of the tradition, disregarding the rest of the process. Thus followers of this watered-down message only become interested in getting a better body. This has left them susceptible to the power of their egos, and causes them to favor their own interpretation of how to practice postures ("I like the *x* system better than the *y* system"). Yet another house has been divided.

When he set forth the Eightfold Path, Patanjali provided a path by which we could let go of our suffering in the material world. Through this path, we may find peace and fully realize the perfection of our spirit. Though he outlined the abstentions and observations as the foundation for this work, the remaining six steps are proactive techniques to be employed every day. An athlete must eat and sleep in a way that prepares his body for optimal performance, but he must also train his body to compete. Similarly, Patanjali teaches us that after shaping our lives around the abstentions and observations, we must prepare our bodies and minds to be available for self-realization.

The abstentions and observations come before the study of posture because committing to these behaviors helps ground us in our intentions for the practice. Then, when it's time to move on to postures, our egos are less likely to mistake physical benefits as the entire path or as a means to compete with ourselves or others. Though they tone the body and make us look healthier, they are simply the third of eight steps. Ultimately, we use postures to make our bodies strong and flexible enough to pursue the remaining five steps—which require sitting for extended periods.

What Is a Posture?

When Yoga was developed over five thousand years ago, one of the main paths was sitting for extended periods in concentration and meditation. The sages immersed in this process came to realize that they needed great health and stamina if they were to sit still. They began to notice that the animals around them stretched after lying down for a while. They soon realized that if they stretched and strengthened their bodies like the animals did, they could sit in greater comfort.

Thousands of years later, Patanjali outlined the next step after the observations as *asana,* which he defined as a steady, comfortable seat. He had little else to say on the matter.

By a steady, comfortable seat, Patanjali referred to what we call the lotus posture: an upright seated position with legs crossed for maximum stability. During Patanjali's time, people didn't live like we do. They didn't sit on couches or eat ice cream and potato chips, so their bodies were more open and flexible than ours. When people sat, they sat on the ground. It is likely that Patanjali gave little explanation of posture because getting into a steady, comfortable seat was far easier and more natural than it is now.

In the fifteenth century, the sage Swami Swatmarama authored what we know as the Hatha Yoga Pradipika. In this document, he outlined several practices related to Patanjali's Eightfold Path as well as other aspects of the Yoga tradition. This document described a handful of postures to be used for meditation and other higher practices. It is considered the oldest existing document describing what we now know as hatha Yoga, which includes breathing techniques, purification techniques, and what we call postures.

Postures are physical positions that emulate animals and other shapes; these shapes give us flexibility and strength, thus facilitating extended periods of sitting. This relatively simple part of the Yogic system was expanded in the last century to include hundreds of positions that came from hundreds of different teachers. Some manuals include over a thousand postures. With the commercialization of Yoga, this information has now been packaged by many schools into books, videos, classes, workshops, retreats, and training programs. Some people have branded postures after themselves, and some of those people have even sued for their right to own the sequences they practice. Though postures are a valid part of Yoga, to reinvent them as belonging to a person or brand only perpetuates a material attachment to the physical realm. It will keep our collective house divided, rather than giving us an opportunity to celebrate the union of body, mind, and spirit, as this system was intended. Postures will ultimately open the body and mind and make them more flexible, but so will eating less, eating natural food, not eating late, and being less emotional.

A glow stick has to be shaken only once before it is used. Once our bodies are open enough to sit for a long time in that steady, comfortable seat that Patanjali wrote about, we no longer need to do postures. The body no longer needs to be shaken—so to speak—for, like the glow stick, it already radiates light.

A Physical Practice in the Three Realms

By now you're probably familiar with the progression from body to mind and then to spirit. Relating to Yogic practices in this way can help us determine where we are on our journey at any given point in our lives. But how do we relate the practice of postures—a primarily physical practice—to the three realms?

The main point of practicing postures is to make the body stronger and more flexible so that we may sit still for lengthy periods. When we practice postures over a long time, though, we must practice in a way that reflects what our bodies need in that chapter of our lives. We can use the realms of body, mind, and spirit to assess where we are in our bodies and how we will benefit from practicing postures—or not practicing them.

The Body: A Physical Practice in a Physical Realm

If everyone's body were the same, we would all benefit from strengthening and stretching in the same way. Each person would practice the same postures for the same amount of time. This is not the case. Some people are particularly flexible in their hamstrings but have tight shoulders. Some people are thin and have hypermobile joints, while others are obese and barely able to move at all.

People who haven't pursued a structured physical discipline often lack a basic awareness of what their body can and can't do. They don't know if their hamstrings or their shoulders are more flexible. Though they could probably guess whether they're able to touch their toes, they haven't tried it recently. The initial step of exploring postures is to develop an awareness of such things, which will lead to greater physical capacity. In the realm of the body, practicing postures allows us to tune in to a part of ourselves that may have gone unattended.

The Mind: Postures and the Curse of the Ego

The ego runs rampant in any situation where participants demonstrate a range of abilities. It's what makes us feel competitive when playing sports, or defeated when we place last in a talent show. Unfortunately, this is apparent in the Western Yoga community. People in the Yoga world often call themselves advanced because they can do poses that other people can't do. Some even think this adds to their spiritual presence. If it were really true that more bendy people had greater spiritual presence, the performers from Cirque du Soleil would be the most spiritually present people in the world. Some of those practitioners—as well as circus performers and contortionists—may very well be in close touch with their spirit. But thinking that flexibility validates one's spiritual quest is really just a trick of the ego. It is a distortion of the mind.

When working in the realm of the body, we become aware of our bodies; in the realm of the mind, we become aware of what we think and feel about our bodies. In the realm of the body, we might say to ourselves, "Oh, when I bend over to touch my toes, I only go halfway down." We didn't have that information, and now we do. But when we say to ourselves, "I can't touch my toes, and that makes me a total, inflexible loser," or "I can balance on my forearms while my feet rest on my head, and this makes me a great Yoga practitioner," we have work to do in the realm of the mind.

What does this work entail? The mental work in postures centers on taking note of where the body is in any given moment and then doing what needs to be done *to serve the body's ability to sustain higher practices along the Yogic path.* This means that if you have particularly flexible shoulders but tight hamstrings, you practice postures to build stability and strength around the shoulder joints and open and lengthen the hamstrings. If you have a history of dancing or competitive gymnastics and have always used your body for exhibition, a mental practice of postures will serve you as you work with your body to attain greater health—especially if you have injuries. Though your work with postures in the realm of the mind is ultimately going to develop your health and well-being—a physical benefit—it will also help you free yourself from the ego. Practicing in this realm will help you sit for extended periods—regardless of what your body could do before you began.

The Spirit: Letting Go of the Physical

When exploring the state of your body by practicing postures, you may find that you're particularly flexible and strong. You may find that you can practice postures for three hours straight and not feel fatigued. But can you then sit upright and remain this way for two hours? Can you simply sit there and breathe without feeling the slightest discomfort from this sustained period of stillness? If you can sit for a third hour and still not feel any discomfort, then you may no longer need postures to continue on your way toward self-realization.

If practicing postures in the realm of the mind challenges us to let go of our feelings about the state of our bodies, practicing postures in the realm of the spirit challenges us to let go of the discipline of postures altogether. Since the purpose of postures is to prepare yourself to sit, they have done their job when sitting in lotus posture is no longer difficult. Sitting like this will prepare you for higher practices, such as breathing, concentration, and meditation. These are the tools that will help you fully realize the perfection of your spirit.

The Plan

As I noted earlier, the Hatha Yoga Pradipika outlines only a handful of postures; the remainder have been formally organized and cataloged in the more recent past. Over the eight weeks in which you will be building a posture practice through the One Plan, you will explore some positions from the Hatha Yoga Pradipika and others that come from more recent times.

The postures that make up the sequences outlined in this plan move the body in nine ways. When you incorporate these nine actions into one cohesive practice, you will have a complete system for building physical health:

GROUNDING

WARMING

STRENGTHENING

FORWARD BENDING

BACKWARD BENDING

BALANCING

INVERTING

TWISTING

HIP OPENING

Each posture will help you practice at least one of these areas, and likely secondary areas as well. For example, one reason for the popularity of Downward-Facing Dog is that it strengthens the body but also bends it forward and inverts it. The sequences commit you to the nine areas in a particular order (after all, warming up at the end of the sequence would be useless). But regardless of what a posture is designed to do, you are the only one who knows what is happening in your own body. Though the postures and sequences that follow will help you open up, it is ultimately up to you to determine if your shoulders, hamstrings, or other parts of the body need to be worked on in certain ways. Ultimately, your purpose is to listen to your body and determine what it needs in any given moment.

The Postures

Here in the One Plan, you will have the opportunity to practice thirty-five postures, with an additional three that serve as variations on how to sit for the higher practices. These postures strengthen and stretch the body in every essential way and direction, and practicing them will help you achieve balance and endurance in the body. I provide a general description of each posture, organized by the primary areas served. When applicable, I also note secondary benefits. Some postures include variations, which can allow for less flexibility in the early stages of practice or be can pursued as a continuation of the earlier practices. What is most important, though, is to practice the continuation postures only after you experience comfort in the earlier ones. Visit my website at yogicameron.com/oneplan to download instructions on how to practice each posture.

Grounding Postures

When entering or finishing a physical practice, it is helpful to center the mind and allow several moments of preparation for whatever is to come next.

MOUNTAIN POSE *(Tadasana)*

This posture allows us to center ourselves and remind ourselves of our intentions for our practice. Secondary action: *balancing*

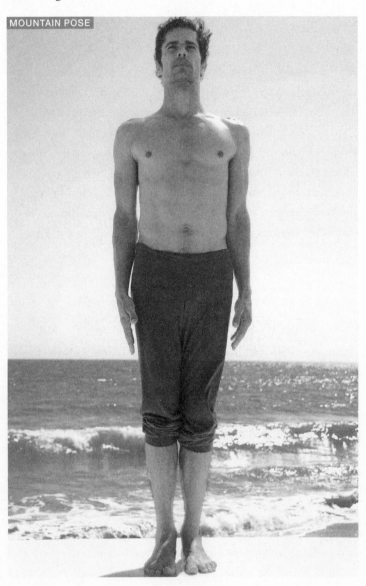

MOUNTAIN POSE

HERO'S POSE (*Virasana*)

This posture also promotes centering. An early variation is to place blankets under the shins to create space for less flexible feet. A continuation is to allow the pelvis to lower between the feet, lower the torso back, and rest on the elbows or all the way onto the back. Secondary actions: *hip opening (with variation), backward bending (with variation)*

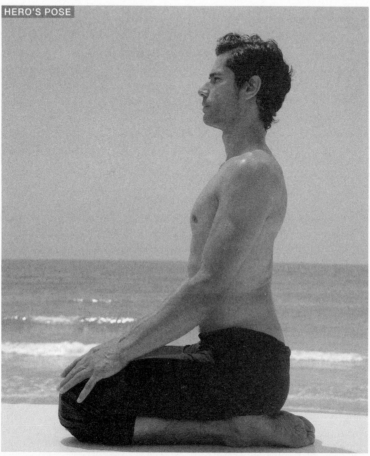

HERO'S POSE

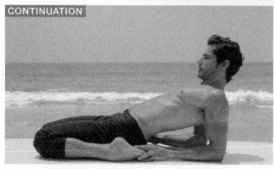

CONTINUATION

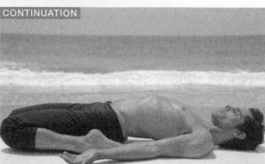

CONTINUATION

CORPSE POSE *(Savasana)*

This posture is typically practiced at the end of a sequence to release tension that may have accumulated during practice.

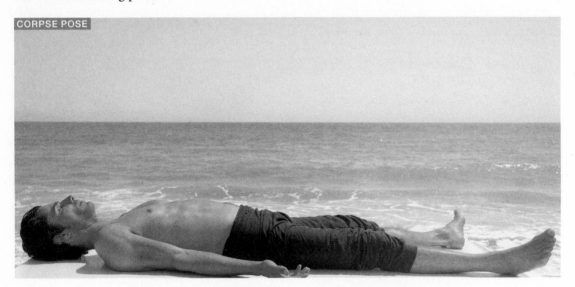

CORPSE POSE

Warming Postures

Early on in a posture practice, the body can be very stiff and cold—especially when you practice soon after waking. These postures are helpful for warming up the body.

CAT/COW *(Marjariasana/Bitilasana)*

These two postures warm up the spine and open the front and back of the body. They are to be practiced in a back-and-forth manner, several seconds at a time. Secondary actions: *forward bending, backward bending*

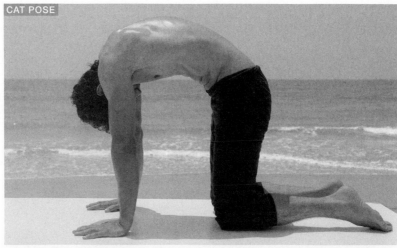

CAT POSE

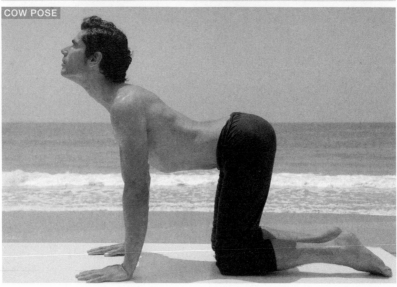

COW POSE

Strengthening Postures

Sitting for prolonged periods requires not only flexibility but strength and stamina. Strong muscles provide greater support of the body's frame, which in turn keeps the joints protected. Some postures will help you find greater strength so as to develop better endurance.

DOWNWARD-FACING DOG *(Adho Mukha Svanasana)*

This is one of the best-known postures and features prominently throughout the sequences presented in the One Plan because of its varied benefits. Secondary actions: *warming, forward bending, inverting*

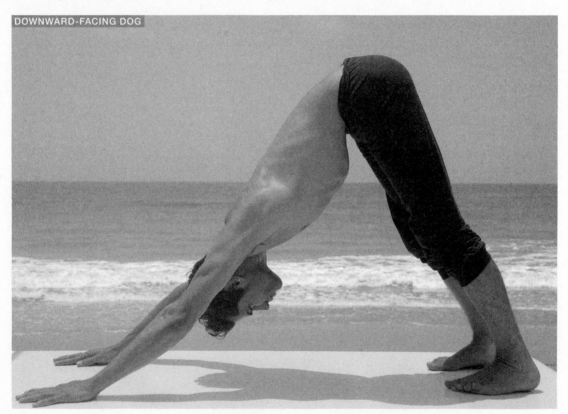

DOWNWARD-FACING DOG

WARRIOR POSE *(Virabhadrasana)*

This series of postures creates strength in the lower body and spine, as well as warming up the body. Variations include Warrior 1, Warrior 2, and Warrior 3. Secondary actions: *warming, hip opening*

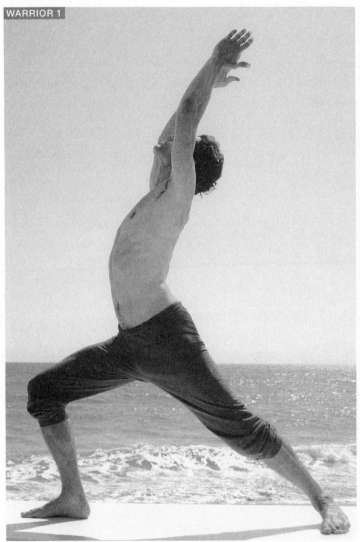

WARRIOR 1

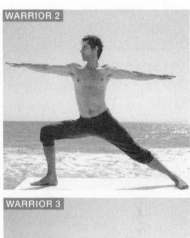

WARRIOR 2

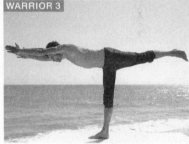

WARRIOR 3

Forward Bending Postures

The back of the body (the back, the buttocks, and the backs of the legs) has many muscle groups in need of lengthening. Some postures focus on opening these muscle groups.

CHILD'S POSE *(Balasana)*

This pose not only opens the back but serves as a way to regroup after more rigorous postures. An early variation is to support the forehead with a block, cushion, or blanket if the head is unable to rest on the ground. Secondary action: *grounding*

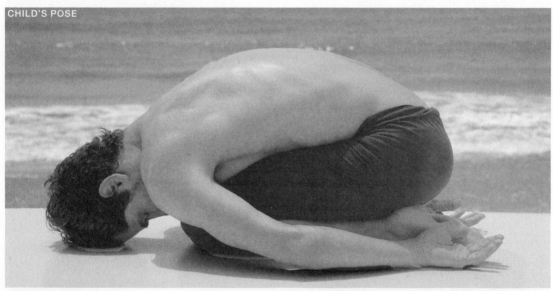

CHILD'S POSE

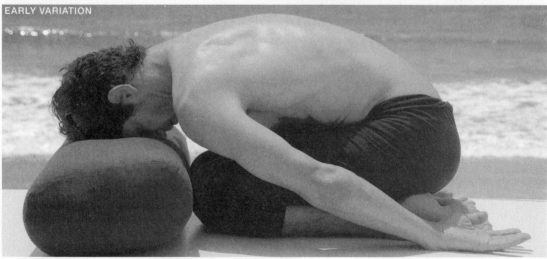

EARLY VARIATION

STANDING FORWARD BEND *(Uttanasana)*

This posture opens the hamstrings and buttocks. Be sure to warm up before practicing this posture. An early variation is to bend the knees slightly. Secondary actions: *inverting, grounding*

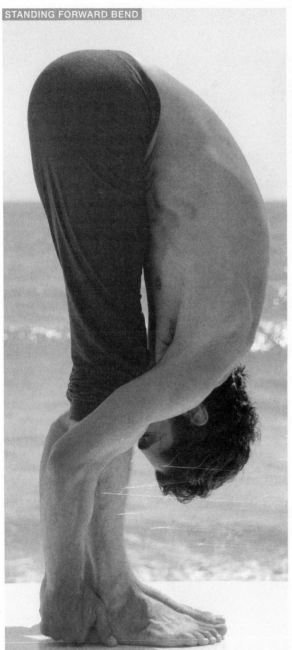

STANDING FORWARD BEND

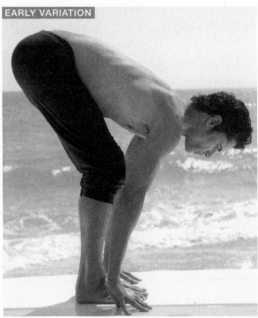

EARLY VARIATION

PYRAMID POSE *(Parsvottanasana)*

This posture provides fairly intense stretching of the back and the backs of the legs. An early variation is to support the hands on blocks. A continuation is to twist the torso and place one hand on the outside of the opposite foot. Secondary action: *hip opening, twisting (with continuation)*

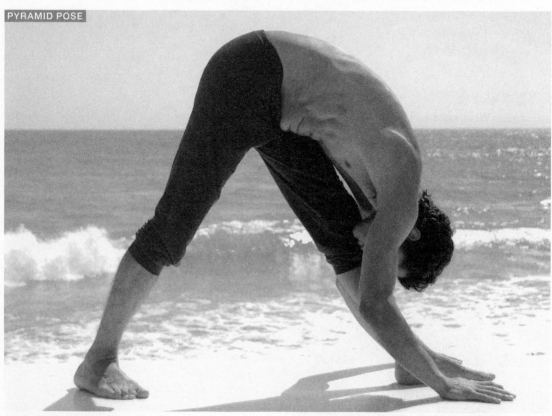

PYRAMID POSE

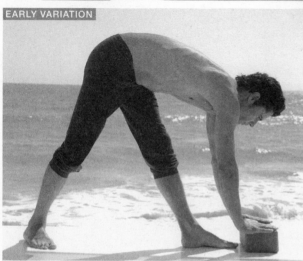

EARLY VARIATION

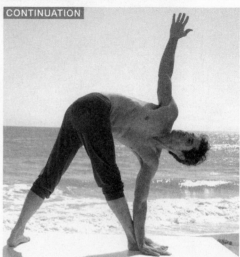

CONTINUATION

PLOUGH POSE *(Halasana)*

This posture in its full form provides an intense opening of the entire back. An early variation is to support the feet on a chair or other raised surface. A continuation is to lower the knees to either side of the ears *(Karnapidasana)*. Secondary action: *inverting*

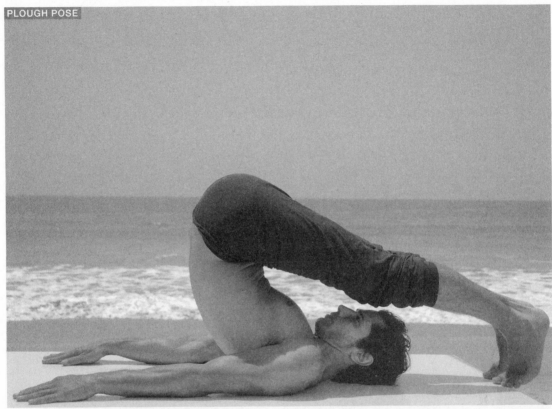

PLOUGH POSE

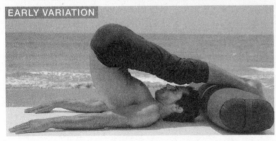

EARLY VARIATION

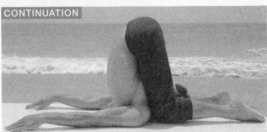

CONTINUATION

HEAD TO KNEE POSE *(Janu Sirsasana)*

This posture stretches one hamstring at a time. An early variation is to raise the pelvis on blankets. A continuation is to twist the body sideways and extend the side of the torso. Secondary actions: *grounding, twisting (with continuation)*

HEAD TO KNEE POSE
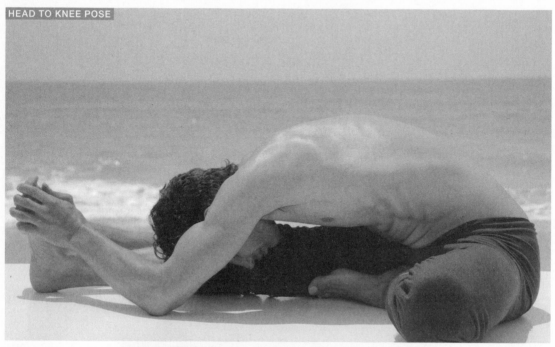

EARLY VARIATION
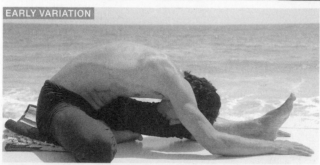

CONTINUATION
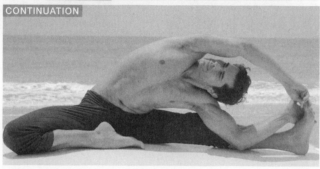

SEATED FORWARD BEND *(Paschimottanasana)*

This posture provides a more intense opening of the hamstrings, as well as opening up the entire back. An early variation is to raise the pelvis on blankets. Secondary action: *grounding*

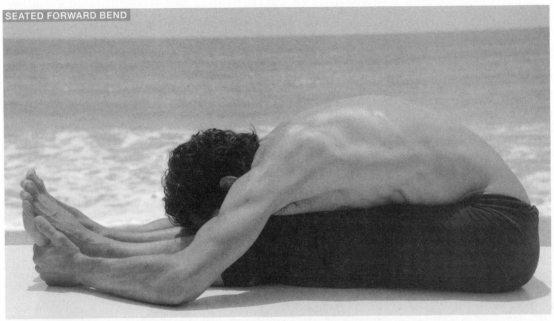
SEATED FORWARD BEND

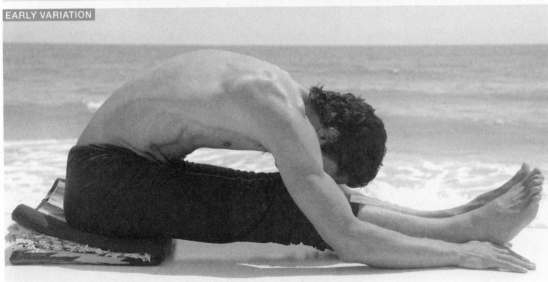
EARLY VARIATION

Backward Bending Postures

The front of the body (the chest, the abdomen, and the fronts of the legs) has many muscle groups. Using postures to bend backward opens these muscle groups and strengthens the spine for prolonged periods of sitting.

COBRA POSE *(Bhujangasana)*

The basic posture provides gentle bending of the back by keeping the torso close to the ground. In the continuation, the upright torso provides full-on bending of the back. Secondary action: *strengthening*

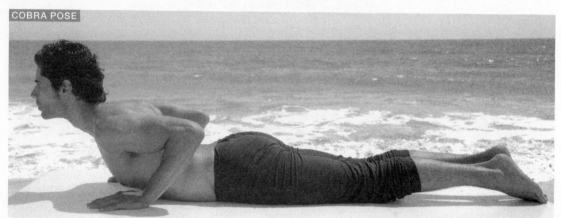
COBRA POSE

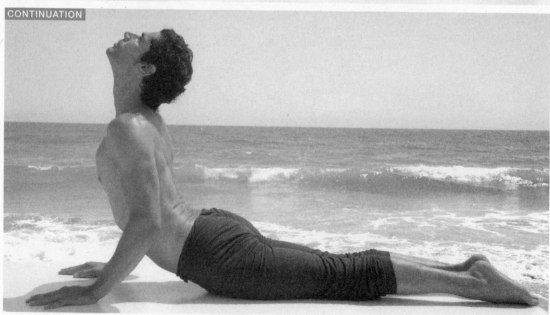
CONTINUATION

BRIDGE POSE *(Setu Bandha Sarvangasana)*

This posture is a gentle way to begin a backward bending practice. An early variation is to support the pelvis with a block. Secondary actions: *strengthening, inverting*

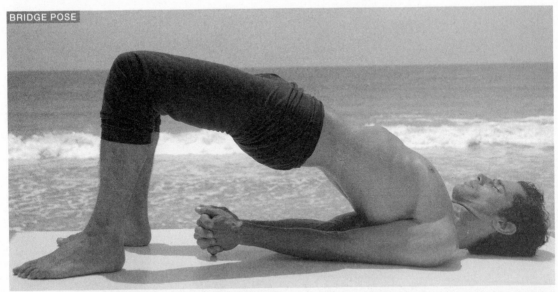

BRIDGE POSE

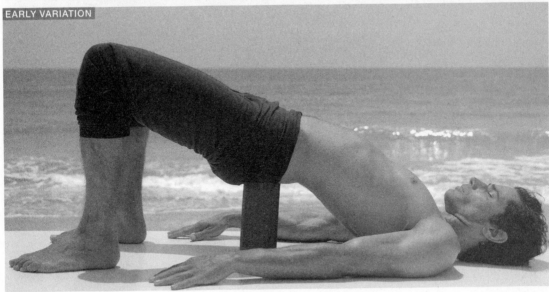

EARLY VARIATION

BOW POSE *(Dhanurasana)*

This posture is equal parts backward bending and strengthening, as much effort is required to raise the body off the ground. Secondary action: *strengthening*

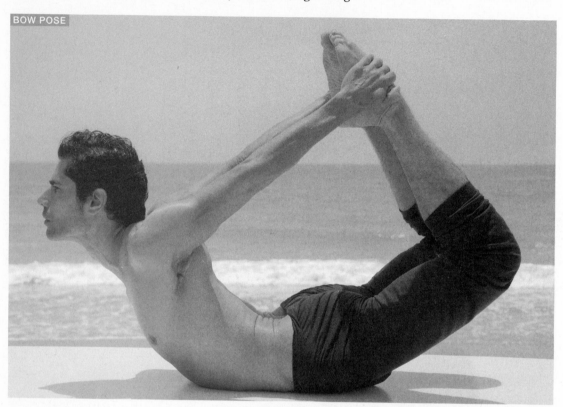

BOW POSE

UPWARD-FACING BOW *(Urdvha Dhanurasana)*

This posture provides an intense backward bend. It is commonly practiced after a gentler backward bending practice has already been explored (such as Bridge Pose). Secondary actions: *strengthening, inverting*

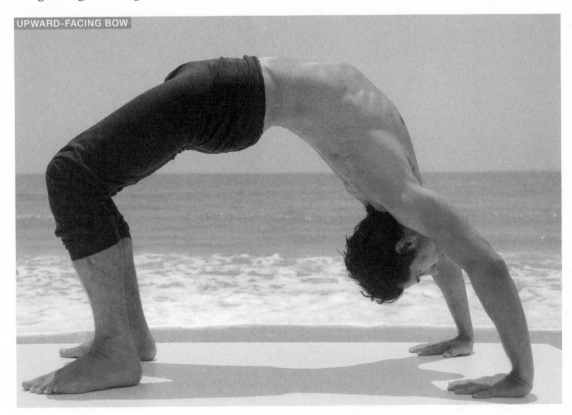

UPWARD-FACING BOW

LOCUST POSE (*Salabasana*)

This posture can be a strong backward bend, depending on the depth to which it is practiced. An early variation is to lift the torso and legs equally off the ground. Secondary action: *strengthening*

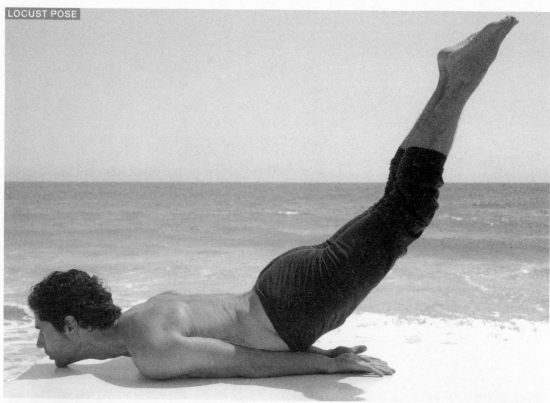

LOCUST POSE

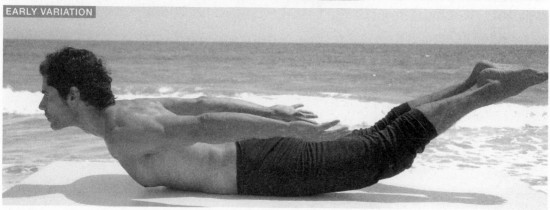

EARLY VARIATION

FISH POSE *(Matsyasana)*

This backward bending posture is of great benefit to the throat and respiratory system. A continuation is to cross the legs in lotus posture and grasp the toes.

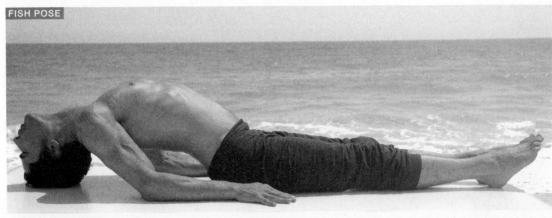

FISH POSE

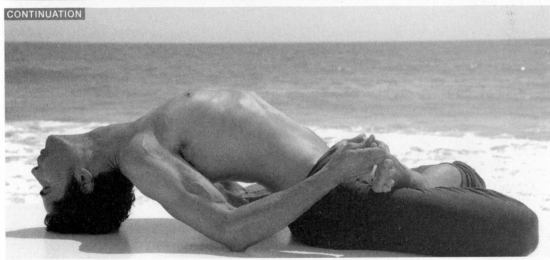

CONTINUATION

Balancing Postures

If you stood on one leg, you'd probably be able to keep your balance pretty well. But if you stood on one leg with your eyes closed, you'd likely fall over. This happens because physical balance is heavily influenced by activity in the mind. The reverse is also true: postures that help you find physical balance have a calming effect on the mind.

TREE POSE *(Vrksasana)*

This posture provides an opportunity to balance and fosters greater focus and presence. An early variation is to place the lifted foot against the ankle or calf. A continuation is to raise the arms and head upward. Secondary action: *hip opening*

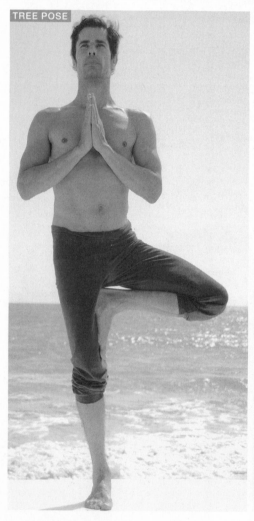

TREE POSE

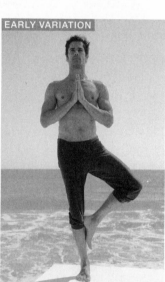

EARLY VARIATION

EARLY VARIATION

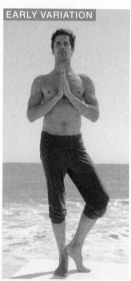

CONTINUATION

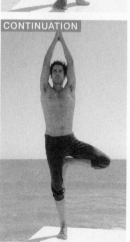

CRANE POSE *(Bakasana)*

This posture, like many arm balances, requires tremendous focus and a willingness to overcome fear. An early variation is to rest the knees on the outsides of the arms. Secondary actions: *strengthening, warming, forward bending*

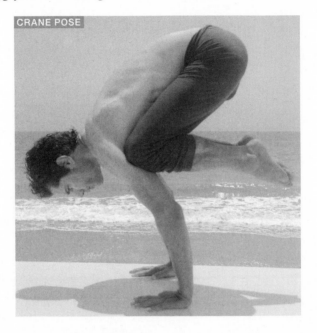

CRANE POSE

EIGHT ANGLE POSE *(Ashtavakrasana)*

This posture, like Crane Pose, is an ambitious exploration of balance and focus. Secondary actions: *strengthening, warming, twisting*

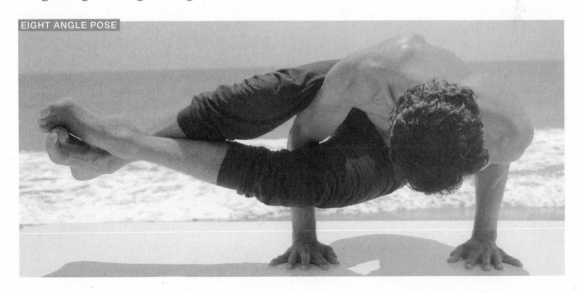

EIGHT ANGLE POSE

PEACOCK POSE *(Mayurasana)*

This posture requires balance and focus but has a therapeutic impact on the digestive system. A continuation is to cross the legs in Lotus position before balancing. Secondary actions: *strengthening, warming*

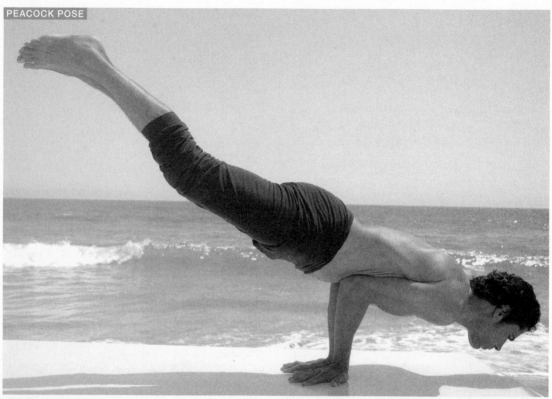

PEACOCK POSE

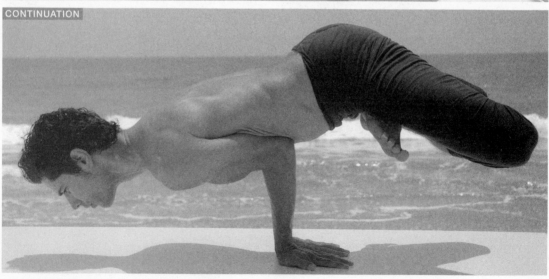

CONTINUATION

Inverting Postures

Between sitting and standing, we spend much of our lives right side up. Inverted postures increase blood circulation to areas that otherwise have gravity working against them, particularly the brain. Some postures invert the body so that the head is at a lower level than the pelvis.

LEGS UP THE WALL *(Viparita Karani)*

This posture creates a gentle inversion in which the raised legs reverse the circulation of the blood without raising the pelvis above the head. It is also possible to practice without a wall by simply raising the legs into the air. Secondary action: *grounding*

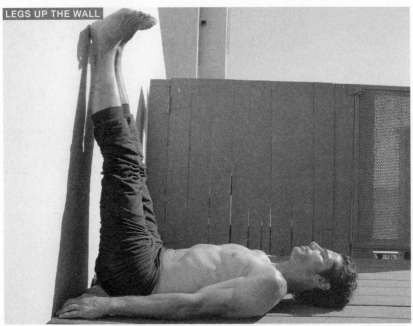

LEGS UP THE WALL

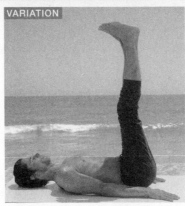

VARIATION

SHOULDER STAND *(Salamba Sarvangasana)*

This inversion is a continuation of the preceding one and can strain the neck if not practiced correctly. A further continuation is to cross the legs in lotus position while in the posture.
Secondary action: *forward bending*

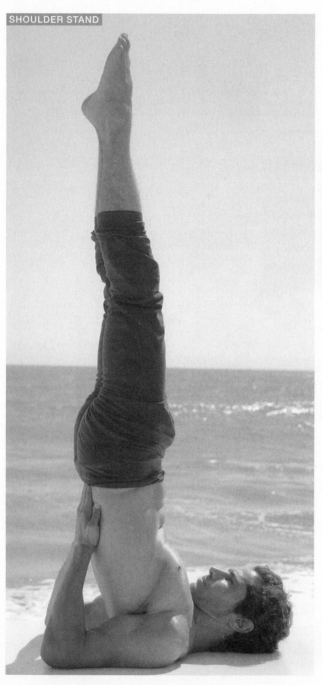

SHOULDER STAND

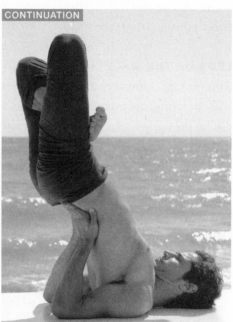

CONTINUATION

HEADSTAND *(Sirsasana)*

A headstand achieves nearly total inversion of the body. It is particularly important to avoid kicking up into Headstand; instead, lift the legs with precision and control. A continuation is the tripod Headstand. Secondary actions: *balancing, strengthening*

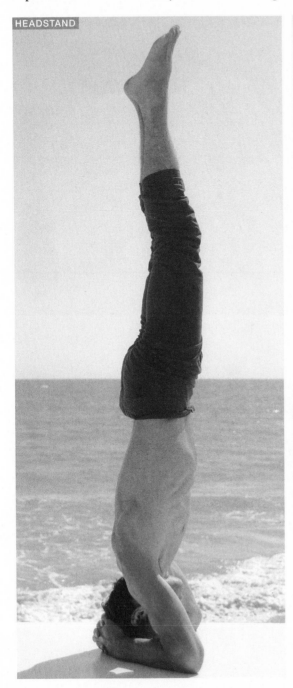

HEADSTAND

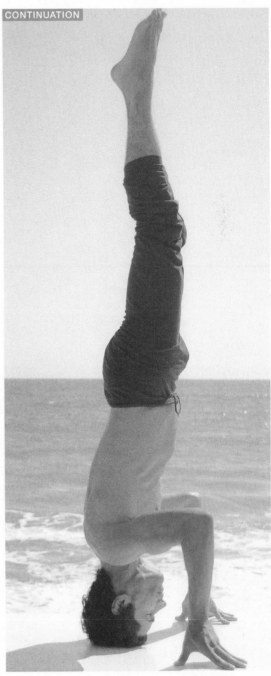

CONTINUATION

HANDSTAND *(Adho Mukha Vrksasana)*

This posture requires total commitment. It is safest to begin practicing with the support of a wall. An early variation is to practice a modified handstand by bending the legs to form an *L*-shape with the feet leaning against a wall. Secondary actions: *balancing, strengthening*

HANDSTAND

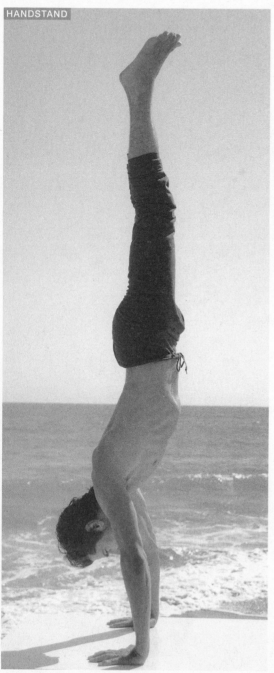

EARLY VARIATION

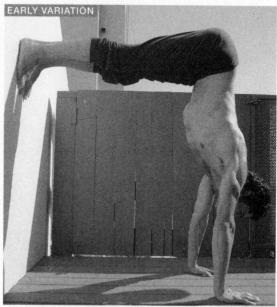

EARLY VARIATION

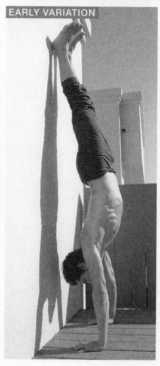

Twisting Postures

Twisting the torso can have a therapeutic effect, as this squeezes the organs, aiding detoxification. Twisting the body also strengthens and stretches associated muscle groups.

SUPINE SPINAL TWIST *(Supta Matsyendrasana)*

This gentle twisting posture provides the benefits of twisting the torso without requiring the strength involved in upright twisting postures. A continuation is to cross the legs before twisting. Secondary action: *grounding*

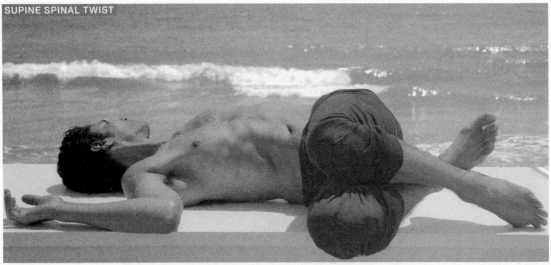

SUPINE SPINAL TWIST

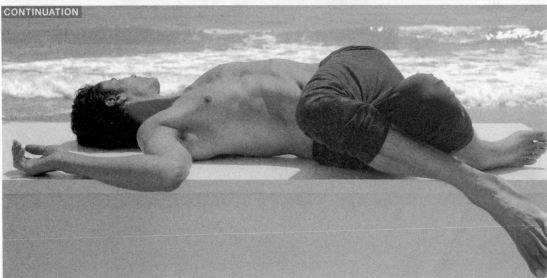

CONTINUATION

HALF LORD OF THE FISHES POSE *(Ardha Matsyendrasana)*

This posture twists the body to its maximum capacity. An early variation is to extend the bottom leg. Secondary action: *hip opening*

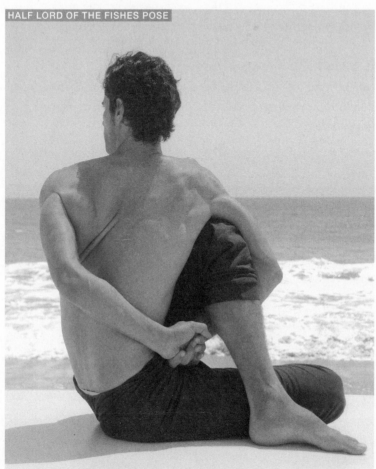

HALF LORD OF THE FISHES POSE

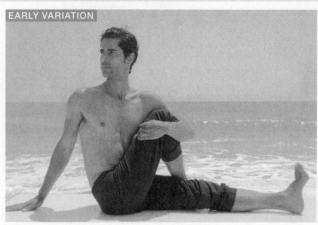

EARLY VARIATION

EXTENDED SIDE ANGLE POSE *(Utthita Parsvakonasana)*

This posture, in addition to twisting the body, stretches the entire side of the torso. Early variations include resting the lower forearm on the thigh of the bent leg and placing the lower hand on the inside of the front foot. A continuation is to bind the hands after wrapping the arms around the bent leg. Secondary actions: *hip opening, strengthening, balancing (for continuation)*

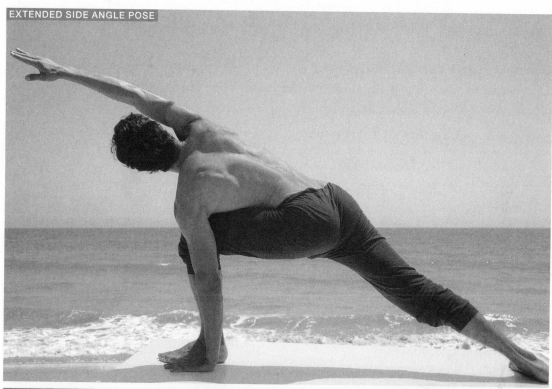

EXTENDED SIDE ANGLE POSE

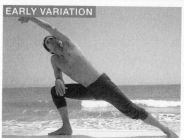

EARLY VARIATION

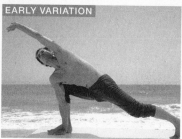

EARLY VARIATION

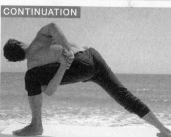

CONTINUATION

Hip Opening Postures

The femurs, or thighbones, connect to the pelvis through what we commonly call hip joints. These ball-and-socket joints are surrounded by a complex of muscles, tendons, and ligaments that often tighten up and prevent us from sitting upright in comfort. Hip opening postures open the muscles and connective tissue of the hips and thus directly prepare you for sitting positions.

LOW CRESCENT LUNGE *(Anjaneyasana)*

This posture opens the hip flexors in the front of the pelvis. An early variation is to rest your arms on your bent leg and hold the spine upright. Secondary actions: *back bending, balancing*

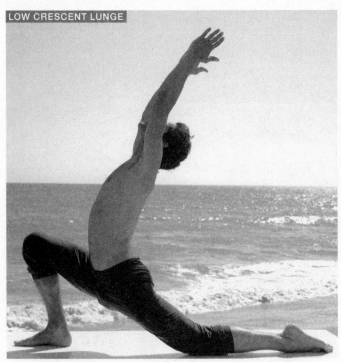

LOW CRESCENT LUNGE

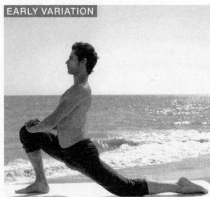

EARLY VARIATION

BUTTERFLY *(Baddha Konasana)*

This posture, formally known as Bound Angle Pose, opens the inner groin muscles and surrounding muscle systems. An early variation is to raise the pelvis with a cushion or some blankets. A continuation is to bend the torso forward over the legs. Secondary action: *forward bending (with continuation)*

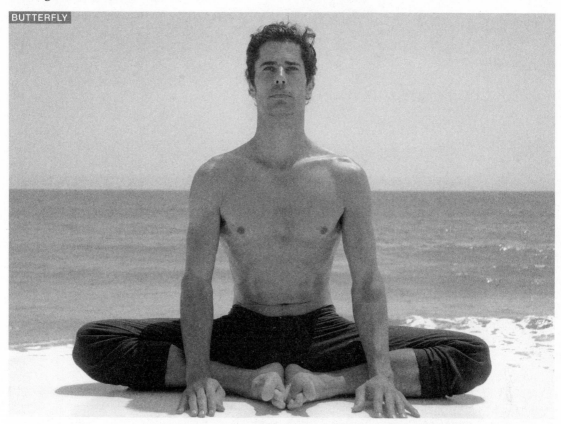

BUTTERFLY

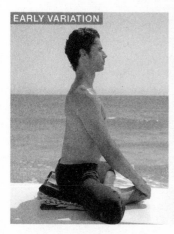

EARLY VARIATION

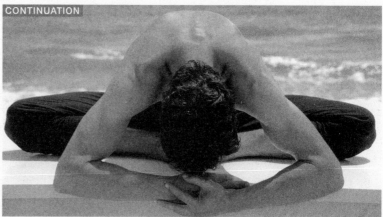

CONTINUATION

BABY CRADLE POSE

This posture gently opens the hips without risking injury to nearby joints like the knees. An early variation is to extend the bottom leg forward.

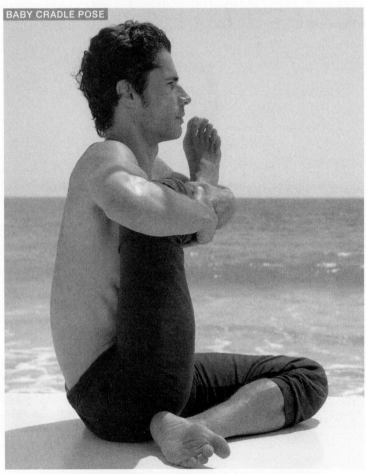

BABY CRADLE POSE

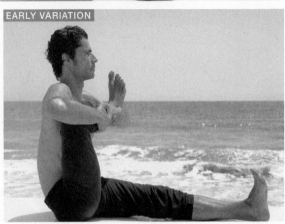

EARLY VARIATION

THREAD THE NEEDLE

This posture provides external rotation and flexion of the hip joint, giving multiple benefits as a hip opener. Secondary action: *forward bending*

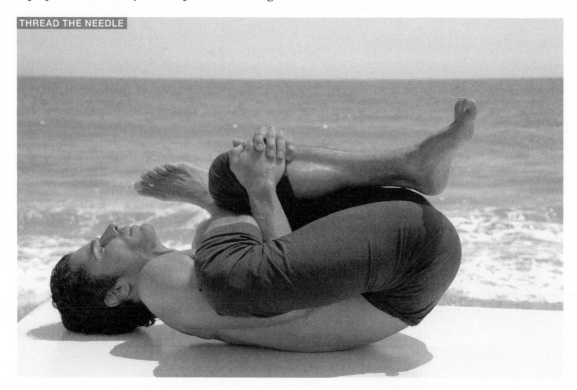

THREAD THE NEEDLE

HALF BOUND LOTUS SEATED FORWARD BEND

(Ardha Baddha Padma Paschimottanasana)

This posture opens the hips in direct preparation for Lotus Pose. An early variation is to remain upright. Secondary actions: *forward bending, twisting*

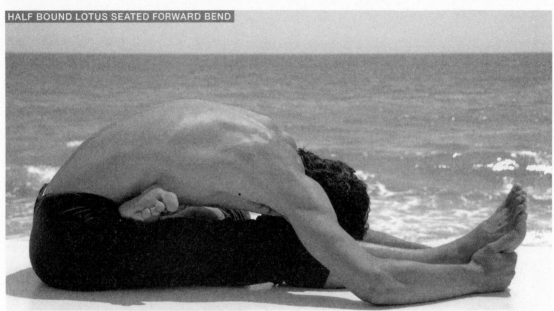

HALF BOUND LOTUS SEATED FORWARD BEND

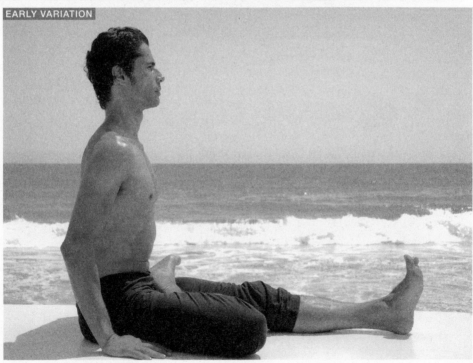

EARLY VARIATION

COW FACE POSE *(Gomukhasana)*

This involved posture is named for its likeness to the face of a cow, and provides significant hip opening as well as opening of the arms and shoulders. A continuation is to bend forward.

Secondary action: *forward bending (with variation)*

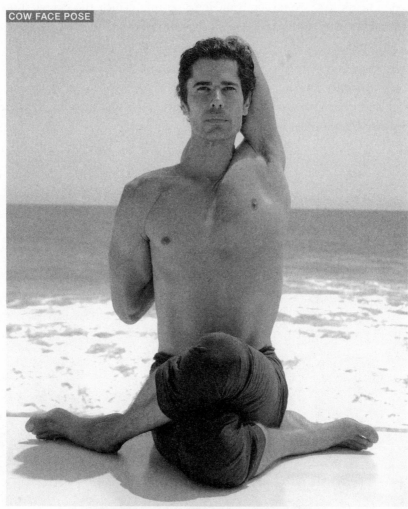

COW FACE POSE

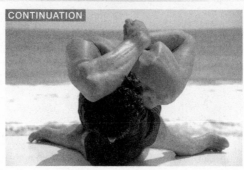

CONTINUATION

Sitting Postures

Sitting with an upright spine provides us with the most alert and focused way to begin developing higher practices. The ultimate expression is the lotus posture, which allows practitioners to remain upright while firmly anchoring themselves with their crossed legs. We can get there by practicing gentler sitting postures.

EASY POSE *(Sukhasana)*

This is the most basic seated posture. It can be made more accessible by supporting the pelvis with a cushion, blankets, or some other firm support.

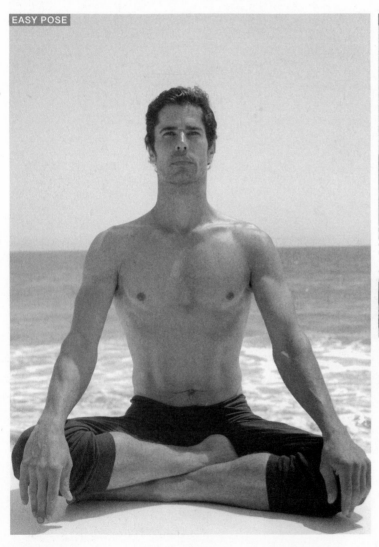

EASY POSE

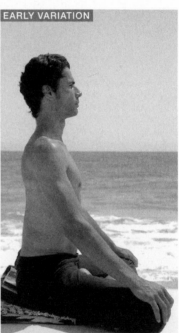

EARLY VARIATION

ADEPT POSE *(Siddhasana)*

This more involved seated posture allows the knees to rest on the ground, improving stability. It too can be made more accessible by adding support under the pelvis.

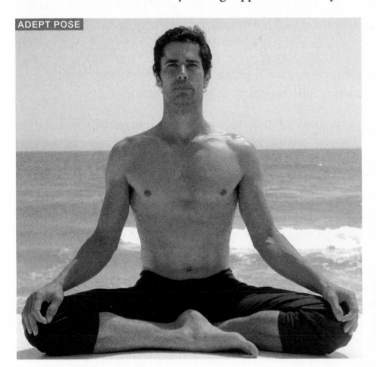

ADEPT POSE

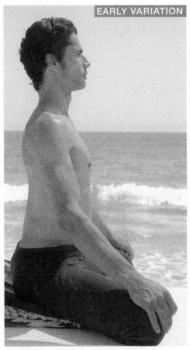

EARLY VARIATION

LOTUS POSE *(Padmasana)*

This posture, which is the ultimate goal of studying Yoga postures, provides the most stable position for sitting with an upright spine over extended periods. The leg position can be incorporated as variations on other postures to intensify the exploration and better prepare the practitioner for long periods in the seated version.

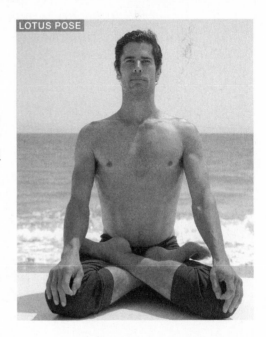

LOTUS POSE

When practicing these and other Yoga postures, always keep the following guidelines in mind:

- *Above all else,* breathe in and out through the nose as you practice each posture. Without the breath, you will undermine your well-being and balance.

- Practice these routines on a Yoga mat or wood floor to maintain the necessary traction. Other surfaces might cause you to slip.

- The routines outlined below include suggested time guidelines. These suggestions may be adapted to your needs.

- If you tend to feel scattered, spacey, and distracted, and you determined from the quiz you took during Weeks 17–18 that you have a lot of Vata energy, practice grounding postures for longer periods, forward bending postures for longer periods, and balancing postures for shorter periods.

- If you tend to be irritable and impatient, you sweat profusely, and you determined from the quiz in Weeks 17–18 that you have a lot of Pitta energy, practice grounding postures for longer periods and strengthening postures for shorter periods.

- If you tend to feel sluggish and lethargic, it's difficult for you to move, and you determined from the quiz in Weeks 17–18 that you have a lot of Kapha energy, practice grounding postures for shorter periods, strengthening postures for longer periods, and balancing postures for longer periods.

The Realm of the Body

The primary purpose of exploring postures in the realm of the body is to develop greater awareness of what the body can and can't do. This is important information, as stiff or unaccommodating bodies are far more prone to injury than bodies that have been trained in a disciplined and balanced way. If you lead a sedentary life or you participate in rigorous physical activities that leave the body tight and prone to injury (such as bodybuilding or American football), you are likely unaware of your body's limits in practicing postures. You will benefit from practicing postures in this realm if you need to take a first step toward tuning in to your body.

Over the next eight weeks, your task is to gradually build up a sequence of fifteen postures. In this realm, you will use props to assist you. This includes using objects like blocks, bolsters, blankets, and straps to help you form the postures in a less demanding way. This assisted approach will allow you to gently work your way into the postures without injuring yourself.

This sequence is to be practiced each morning after you have practiced your purity routine. In this part of your practice, spend seven days with each new version of the sequence. Follow the guidelines below to gradually build up to the full fifteen-posture sequence, which you will practice from the eighth week on.

WEEK 1: Practice Cat/Cow, Downward-Facing Dog (*Adho Mukha Svanasana*), and Child's Pose (*Balasana*). This practice provides a simple way to begin physicalizing your daily routine.

1. Begin on hands and knees and alternate between Cat and Cow for about a minute.

2. Practice Downward-Facing Dog for ten or fifteen seconds.

3. Come into Child's Pose and remain there for twenty or thirty seconds.

4. Repeat Downward-Facing Dog for fifteen or twenty seconds.

5. Come into Child's Pose and remain there for a full minute. Remind yourself to focus on your breathing. As thoughts come up, return your focus to your breath.

WEEK 2: Add Cobra Pose (*Bhujangasana*) to the sequence. This will introduce backward bending into the routine.

1. Begin on hands and knees and alternate between Cat and Cow for about a minute.

2. Practice Downward-Facing Dog for ten or fifteen seconds.

3. Come onto the stomach and practice Cobra Pose for twenty or thirty seconds.

4. Come into Child's Pose and remain there for twenty or thirty seconds.

5. Repeat Downward-Facing Dog for twenty or thirty seconds.

6. Practice Child's Pose again, this time for a full minute.

WEEK 3: Add Low Crescent Lunge (*Anjaneyasana*) to the sequence. This will introduce hip opening into the routine.

1. Begin on hands and knees and alternate between Cat and Cow for about a minute.

2. Practice Downward-Facing Dog for ten or fifteen seconds.

3. Come onto the stomach and practice Cobra Pose for twenty or thirty seconds.

4. Come into Child's Pose and remain there for twenty or thirty seconds.

5. Practice Low Crescent Lunge for fifteen or twenty seconds on each side.

6. Repeat Downward-Facing Dog for twenty or thirty seconds.

7. Practice Child's Pose again, this time for a full minute.

WEEK 4: Add Mountain Pose (*Tadasana*) and Corpse Pose (*Savasana*) to the sequence. This will introduce grounding, which provides a way to settle into the intentions of the routine at the beginning and let go of the routine at the end.

1. Begin in Mountain Pose, with your hands in prayer in front of your chest. Remain there for twenty or thirty seconds.

2. Come to hands and knees and alternate between Cat and Cow for about a minute.

3. Practice Downward-Facing Dog for ten or fifteen seconds.

4. Come onto the stomach and practice Cobra Pose for twenty or thirty seconds.

5. Come into Child's Pose and remain there for twenty or thirty seconds.

6. Practice Low Crescent Lunge for fifteen or twenty seconds on each side.

7. Repeat Downward-Facing Dog for twenty or thirty seconds.

8. Practice Child's Pose again, this time for a full minute.

9. Lie on your back in Corpse Pose, remaining there for at least three minutes. Continue to focus on your breath.

WEEK 5: Add Tree Pose (*Vrksasana*) to the sequence. This will introduce balancing, which is a natural next step after establishing a grounding practice.

1. Begin in Mountain Pose, with your hands in prayer position. Remain there for twenty or thirty seconds.

2. Come to hands and knees and alternate between Cat and Cow for about a minute.

3. Practice Downward-Facing Dog for ten or fifteen seconds.

4. Come onto the stomach and practice Cobra Pose for twenty or thirty seconds.

5. Come into Child's Pose and remain there for twenty or thirty seconds.

6. Practice Low Crescent Lunge for fifteen or twenty seconds on each side.

7. Come to your feet and practice Tree Pose for twenty or thirty seconds on each side.

8. Repeat Downward-Facing Dog for twenty or thirty seconds.

9. Practice Child's Pose again, this time for a full minute.

10. Lie on your back in Corpse Pose, remaining there for at least three minutes.

WEEK 6: Add Legs up the Wall (*Viparita Karani*) and Supine Spinal Twist (*Supta Matsyendrasana*) to the sequence. This will introduce inverting and twisting to the sequence.

1. Begin in Mountain Pose. Remain there for twenty or thirty seconds.

2. Come to hands and knees and alternate between Cat and Cow for about a minute.

3. Practice Downward-Facing Dog for ten or fifteen seconds.

4. Come onto the stomach and practice Cobra Pose for twenty or thirty seconds.

5. Come into Child's Pose and remain there for twenty or thirty seconds.

6. Practice Low Crescent Lunge for fifteen or twenty seconds on each side.

7. Come to your feet and practice Tree Pose for twenty or thirty seconds on each side.

8. Repeat Downward-Facing Dog for twenty or thirty seconds.

9. Practice Child's Pose again, this time for a full minute.

10. Practice Legs up the Wall for a full minute.

11. Practice Spinal Twist for twenty or thirty seconds on each side.

12. Lie on your back in Corpse Pose, remaining there for at least three minutes.

WEEK 7: Add Bridge Pose (*Setu Bandha Sarvangasana*) to the sequence. This provides an additional way to explore back bending.

1. Begin in Mountain Pose. Remain there for twenty or thirty seconds.

2. Come to hands and knees and alternate between Cat and Cow for about a minute.

3. Practice Downward-Facing Dog for ten or fifteen seconds.

4. Come onto the stomach and practice Cobra Pose for twenty or thirty seconds.

5. Come into Child's Pose and remain there for twenty or thirty seconds.

6. Practice Low Crescent Lunge for fifteen or twenty seconds on each side.

7. Come to your feet and practice Tree Pose for twenty or thirty seconds on each side.

8. Lie on your back and practice Bridge Pose for twenty or thirty seconds.

9. Repeat Downward-Facing Dog for twenty or thirty seconds.

10. Practice Child's Pose again, this time for a full minute.

11. Practice Legs up the Wall for a full minute.

12. Practice Spinal Twist for twenty or thirty seconds on each side.

13. Lie on your back in Corpse Pose, remaining there for at least three minutes.

WEEK 8: Add Butterfly (*Baddha Konasana*) to the sequence. This is an additional way to explore hip opening.

1. Begin in Mountain Pose. Remain there for twenty or thirty seconds.

2. Come to hands and knees and alternate between Cat and Cow for about a minute.

3. Practice Downward-Facing Dog for ten or fifteen seconds.

4. Come onto the stomach and practice Cobra Pose for twenty or thirty seconds.

5. Come into Child's Pose and remain there for twenty or thirty seconds.

6. Practice Low Crescent Lunge for fifteen or twenty seconds on each side.

7. Come to your feet and practice Tree Pose for twenty or thirty seconds on each side.

8. Lie on your back and practice Bridge Pose for twenty or thirty seconds.

9. Sit up and practice Butterfly for twenty or thirty seconds.

10. Repeat Downward-Facing Dog for twenty or thirty seconds.

11. Practice Child's Pose again, this time for a full minute.

12. Practice Legs up the Wall for a full minute.

13. Practice Spinal Twist for twenty or thirty seconds on each side.

14. Lie on your back in Corpse Pose, remaining there for at least three minutes.

When you maintain this sequence over a period of several months or even a year, you will start to see your body open into fuller expression of the postures. At first, you may need support under your head when you practice Child's Pose, but eventually your head will completely lower to the ground. Your knees may at first be high above the ground when you're in Butterfly, but eventually they will lower several inches. Not only will you become stronger and healthier, but you will become aware of your body in subtle—and not so subtle—ways.

Tuning in to your body will help you tune into your anatomy and physiology, including taking note of what is happening in your joints and observing the relative ease or dis-ease of your digestion. From this heightened awareness, you will be able to make more informed decisions on how to live well.

The Realm of the Mind

You may already have a flexible body, or you may have practiced postures for years. Because postures are designed to prepare our bodies for extended periods of sitting, the only thing that matters is how well we've prepared ourselves for this task.

Over the eight weeks of practicing postures in the realm of the mind, you will start with a twenty-one-posture sequence that expands the one provided in the eighth week of the realm of the body. Then, for each of the remaining seven weeks, you will experiment with adapting the sequence using postures that are a continuation of the original twenty-one. Sometimes you may find that you're ready for these continuations, and sometimes you'll find that you're better off remaining true to the original postures. You may even want to return to some earlier variations. The real work here, aside from the physical challenges and rigors of the practice itself, is to *practice only postures that you are truly ready for.* If you listen to your ego and set out to practice postures beyond your ability, not only will you be trapped by your mind but you may hurt yourself. You will be ready to move past this realm when you have the physical ability to sit for extended periods without discomfort and you're able to let go of postures as reflections of how advanced, beginner, valid, invalid, spiritual, or nonspiritual you are. And of course, nobody can actually be nonspiritual. We remain spiritual beings—especially after passing out of the body.

The process you will go through over these eight weeks is as follows:

WEEK 1: Practice the twenty-one-posture sequence.

1. Mountain Pose *(Tadasana)*
2. Cat/Cow *(Marjariasana/Bitilasana)*
3. Downward-Facing Dog *(Adho Mukha Svanasana)*
4. Warrior 2 *(Virabhadrasana 2)*
5. Cobra Pose *(Bhujangasana)*
6. Low Crescent Lunge *(Anjaneyasana)*

7. Child's Pose *(Balasana)*

8. Standing Forward Bend *(Uttanasana)*

9. Tree Pose *(Vrksasana)*

10. Hero's Pose *(Virasana)*

11. Bow Pose *(Dhanurasana)*

12. Bridge Pose *(Setu Bandha Sarvangasana)*

13. Fish Pose *(Matsyasana)*

14. Head to Knee Pose *(Janu Sirsasana)*

15. Butterfly *(Baddha Konasana)*

16. Seated Forward Bend *(Paschimottanasana)*

17. Plough Pose *(Halasana)*

18. Shoulder Stand *(Salamba Sarvangasana)*

19. Thread the Needle

20. Half Lord of the Fishes Pose *(Ardha Matsyendrasana)*

21. Corpse Pose *(Savasana)*

WEEK 2: Try replacing Warrior 2 with Extended Side Angle *(Utthita Parsvakonasana)*, Warrior 1 *(Virabhadrasana 1)*, or Warrior 3 *(Virabhadrasana 3)*. When practicing Extended Side Angle, experiment with the three variations.

WEEK 3: Try replacing Standing Forward Bend with Pyramid Pose *(Parsvottanasana)* on each side. If Pyramid Pose feels comfortable, experiment with rotating the torso to practice the revolved variation of Pyramid.

WEEK 4: Try replacing Bow Pose with Locust Pose *(Salabasana)*.

WEEK 5: Try replacing Bridge Pose with Upward-Facing Bow Pose *(Urdvha Dhanurasana)*.

WEEK 6: Try replacing Tree Pose with Crane Pose *(Bakasana)*, Eight Angle Pose *(Ashtavakrasana)*, or Peacock Pose *(Mayurasana)*.

WEEK 7: Try replacing Hero's Pose with Headstand *(Sirsasana)* or Handstand *(Adho Mukha Vrksasana)*.

WEEK 8: Try adding Baby Cradle, Cow Face Pose *(Gomukhasana)*, or Half Bound Lotus Seated Forward Bend *(Ardha Baddha Padma Paschimottanasana)* to the sequence after Thread the Needle.

Now, does this mean that you must practice these continuations instead of the original twenty-one-posture sequence for as long as you practice postures? Of course not. Though practicing these more involved postures will make you stronger and more flexible, you may be years from practicing them as well. The purpose of experimenting during these eight weeks is to help you distinguish between what you are practicing because it's the natural next step of your physical exploration and what you are practicing because of a desire to compete with yourself or others. You may never actually practice Handstand, and that would be okay. What's important is for you to train your mind to accept your physical posture practice for whatever it needs to be in the present moment. This reflects pursuing balance over desire and is true to a Yogic way of thinking.

You may have a posture routine that you already practice, whether because you go to Yoga class on a regular basis or because you practice a routine that you've picked up somewhere. Your work in the realm of the mind can absolutely include this routine instead, but the important thing is to practice it at home in the morning as a setup for the practices that follow. Going to class may get you to be more flexible and energized, but practicing at home will help you build willpower. This practice will lead you to be at one with your inner guru, which will teach you everything you need to know to make postures a balancing experience instead of just a physical exercise. Your perception of yourself will improve, and you will start to communicate with your spirit.

The Realm of the Spirit

The more followers of this path control and train their bodies, the more detached they become from what they can and can't do. You will be ready to practice postures in the realm of the spirit when you are able to sit in lotus posture or an appropriate variation of it (such as Adept Pose, *Siddhasana*) for extended periods of time—and without extensive preparation on any given day. This means that you can simply wake up in the morning, get a few creaks out of the body with a few choice postures, and then be ready to sit.

Should you ever be at this point yourself, a recommended routine is to practice a half dozen postures in the morning that cover most of the areas (a sample sequence is Cat/Cow, Downward-Facing Dog, Bound Extended Side Angle, Upward-Facing Bow, Shoulder Stand, and Corpse) and then assume your position in Lotus. Build your ability to sit in this posture over time. You will then be ready for the remainder of your more subtle practices.

Emerging as a Masterpiece

Many of the practices you will add to your routine from this point on require an ever-increasing commitment of time. The time spent practicing postures is ultimately an investment in improving the quality of the rest of your day. In addition to preparing you to take a steady, comfortable seat, a dedicated posture practice will help your respiration, your circulation, and your other systems to function better. You will return to your natural weight, if being overweight or obese is an issue for you. You will feel healthier and therefore take greater delight in your experiences throughout the day. You will begin to see that there really is a masterpiece within that you are uncovering each and every day you remain committed to this path.

Putting It Together

If you are pursuing this program entirely within the realm of the body, your routine will be as follows:

- Continue your daily purity practices each morning.

- Build up to practicing the thirteen-posture sequence.

- Take herbal tea twice a day to continue building strength and cleanliness.

And remember . . .

- Continue eating half as much processed food and unhealthy substances as you did prior to the program, avoid eating during the last two hours of the day, and release your sexual essence half as often as you did before Week 7. Avoid accumulating more possessions.

- Continue building your nonviolence, truthfulness, nonstealing, and austerity behaviors to the best of your ability. Continue participating in a physical activity that requires presence of mind at least once every two weeks.

- Eat your lunch in silence at least once a week. Go for a brief walk or jog as well.

- Commit some time each day to an act of service toward a family member, a friend, a colleague, or someone else who crosses your path.

- Consider fasting for a day every two weeks.

If you are practicing exclusively in the realm of the mind, your daily practice over these two weeks will look like this:

- Spend ten minutes of your morning repeating the Gayatri Mantra.

- Practice the most beneficial version of the twenty-one-posture sequence given where you are in your body.

- Read the Yoga Sutras or other spiritual material for five minutes before you go to bed.

And remember . . .

- Continue eating natural foods, refrain from eating in the last five hours of the day and after 7 P.M., and continue to have sex in moderation.

- Continue your nonviolence, truthfulness, nonstealing, austerity, and self-study practices, and avoid sexual thoughts. Continue to let go of attachments to people and situations that you are keeping out of fear.

- Continue to take note of your situational desires and create alternate possibilities for your life, and continue to observe your thoughts in emotionally heightened situations. Continue to practice self-surrender in one area of your life.

- Consider fasting for one day each week.

correcting the great mistake

BREATH CONTROL

CLIENTS COME TO ME WITH MANY DIFFERENT AILMENTS. SOME struggle with their energy, while others struggle with their weight. But one of the most common themes is a struggle with breathing. Whether they have asthma or are prone to chronic respiratory ailments like bronchitis, they often consider it their lot in life. Usually they medicate with inhalers and antibiotics. But they are among the few who give breathing a second thought. The problem is that it's not just asthmatics and the chronically congested who are struggling. Most of us struggle because of our breath every day.

One time, I worked with a client who was prone to strong emotions when she talked with others. She initially contacted me because she was overwhelmed with stress. During our first consultation, I asked her how she felt she breathed.

"What do you mean, how do I feel I breathe?" she said, almost irritated by the question. "I breathe in, I breathe out. It's as simple as that, isn't it?"

"And how often do you work on your breathing?" I asked.

"Work on it?" she said. "Why would I work on something that happens naturally?"

I then asked her one more question: "What would happen if you stopped breathing entirely?" At this point, she was probably wondering why she had asked a former supermodel to help her with stress, since these questions were adding to it. "Well, you would die, wouldn't you?" she finally said.

"Maybe," I said, smiling.

"Maybe?" she said, her voice getting tense. "How would I be able to live if I didn't breathe?"

"Well," I said, "I'm sure there have been moments when you didn't."

"Like when?"

I looked at her. "Like right now."

She broke off what had been a rather challenging stare to process this. Sure enough, half a second later, she exhaled loudly. She had been holding her breath for the better part of our conversation.

Though I felt a little naughty for putting her on the spot like that, my purpose was clear: she believed breathing was an involuntary action, and yet being frustrated by my questions caused her enough stress to stop breathing. If breathing were involuntary, then why did she stop doing it? And why was she so agitated by a simple conversation?

Our Mistaken Breaths

My client is like a lot of people. She experienced significant stress in her life and was prone to emotional outbursts. After she expressed embarrassment for her irritation, we explored the questions I had posed. How did she feel she breathed? Poorly. How often did she work on her breathing? Never. And what would happen if she stopped breathing? Well, eventually she would expire, but before that happened, she would probably experience more of the same things: stress, frustration, and troubled emotions.

Her reaction to these questions reflects an underlying problem in our culture. On the whole, we breathe improperly and use the breath only for survival. This undermines our ability to work through stressful situations, temper difficult emotions, and frankly, live long and healthy lives. This issue affects nearly everyone in different ways.

We take frequent breaths. The average human being takes between twelve and twenty breaths per minute, depending on their character. I've worked with clients who breathed even more frequently. Though this may seem like a good range, the truth is that Mother Nature rewards those members of the animal kingdom who take fewer breaths per minute with greater longevity. Field mice take anywhere between eighty and two hundred breaths per minute, and they only live one to three years. The giant tortoise, known for its life span of more than 150 years, only breathes four times per minute. When I'm not practicing Yoga techniques, I take only about six breaths per minute.

We take shallow breaths. Somewhere along the line, we started calling a breath that uses the entire capacity of the lungs a "deep breath." This type of breath involves expansion of the abdomen and a long, sustained inhalation and exhalation. The term *deep breath* is really a misnomer, for when we use the full capacity of our lungs, we're not taking a deep breath—we're simply taking the full breath we're supposed to be taking all the time.

We hold our breath. Whether because we're filled with tension over something bad we fear may happen, or because we're wrapped up in what we're doing and have lost all awareness of ourselves, or because a naughty yogi decides to have some fun with us by asking frustrating questions during a consultation, we often hold our breath.

You may be thinking that plenty of people never give their breath any consideration at all, but they live long enough, endure stress, and get on with their lives. Though improper breathing may keep us alive, it undermines our health and exacerbates our emotions. And if the point of life is to be healthy and happy and to find our spiritual purpose, then just breathing for survival allows us to catch only a tiny glimpse of our potential.

The Breath and Health

It has been said by past yogis that we are allotted a certain number of breaths in a lifetime. By taking frequent breaths, we use up that allotment much quicker and undermine our longevity. When we use our full lung capacity, the lungs become more efficient. Then they are capable of delivering more oxygen to the trillions of cells in the body and can expel all of the toxic impurities from the system. This prevents onset of disease and helps the body and mind function at their peak performance.

Holding the breath has a detrimental impact on our health for the same reasons we need to keep breathing in general. If we habitually hold our breath, we're limiting our respiratory system's ability to keep us disease-free. Does this mean that if we hold our breath for a few moments we're going to die? No, but forgetting to breathe on a regular basis will ultimately deplete the body's oxygen supply, and when this problem is left unchecked, it will cause dysfunction in any number of physiological systems. It will especially compromise the nervous system, which controls our emotions and stress levels.

Scientists have conducted numerous studies of the potential physiological benefits of a breath control practice. One study, published in 2006 by the medical journal *Medical Hypotheses,* suggests that Yogic breathing practices help modulate the nervous system, increase the stabilizing activity of the parasympathetic nervous system, and facilitate alertness and reinvigoration. Another study, published in 2009 by *Annals of the New York Academy of Sciences,* found that breath work induces stress resilience. Studies have repeatedly shown that this type of activity has a measurable impact on the practitioner's health.

We can compare breathing to eating food. If you were to eat nothing but large amounts of junk food, you might continue to go from hungry to satiated and keep yourself alive. You might be overweight, have diabetes, frequently get sick, and never have any energy, but you accept this as the nature of living. But what would happen if one day you started eating natural foods? Suddenly, you would lose weight. You would hardly ever get sick. Thanks to expressions like "you are what you eat," most of us know to associate poor eating habits with an unhealthy life. But how many of us know that "we are what we *breathe*?" How many of us know that breathing frequently and shallowly as well as holding our breath is having as much of an impact as subsisting on snack cakes?

Though it may seem like we live long enough and are healthy enough, we would live even longer, healthier lives if we incorporated beneficial breathing into our routines. Breathing properly leads to less stress and higher functioning of the body's systems, including the nervous system. It is like putting fruits and vegetables into our lungs so that our bodies can achieve peak performance.

The Breath and Emotions

As if it weren't enough that poor breathing shortens our lives and compromises our health, it can also increase emotional upset throughout the day.

Let's say you're at work and your boss is having a particularly bad day. He storms into your office and accuses you of incompetence. He hurls hostility at you in angry pants and grunts. He breathes quickly and shallowly as he spews out his frustration, and your breathing falls into rhythm with his. He's angry, and you've invested in the breathing rhythms produced by that anger. You've been swept away by the emotions of the moment, and you respond with sadness, guilt, fear, or even your own anger. What would have happened if you had maintained a slower, fuller breath throughout the experience? Would he have continued yelling? Maybe. But how would you have felt inside?

When we breathe poorly, we are more susceptible to adverse emotions—particularly when those emotions stem from a contentious encounter. When an angry person is yelling at us, our senses tell us that something bad is happening, and our emotions join in that negativity. But breathing slowly and fully allows us to connect with the calm center of who we are—our spirit—as opposed to the stimulation taken in by our senses. Many people in the West recognize the power of the breath as a source of calm, as when they tell someone who's upset to "slow down and take a deep breath." These people likely don't have much knowledge of the Yogic path, but the teachings are the same.

If the boss comes in to yell at you, maintain slow, full breaths. He might continue his tirade, but because you haven't invested in his angry panting, your senses won't allow his quick breathing to influence your calm and peace. Rather than getting upset, you can simply observe him in his agitated state and let him be. And your calm will beget more calm: you'll probably jolt him out of his tantrum just as quickly as he entered it. Thus you will have helped him find a way out of his misery.

Breath Control

The fourth step on Patanjali's Eightfold Path is *pranayama*. This Sanskrit word refers to controlling the breath to create a beneficial flow of energy throughout the body. Pranayama moves breathing from an involuntary state to a voluntary one. With greater energy flow, our minds remain in a state of balance. Improved balance in the mind leads to better functioning of the body and less intense emotional reactions. When we learn to not just fully use our breath but effectively control it, we feel healthier and more peaceful, and we take a significant step toward ending the suffering that compelled us to seek the Yogic path in the first place.

The Body: Breath Control Enhances Health

The first step in creating a breathing practice is to train the body to breathe more slowly, fully, and consistently. This happens by making a conscious effort to regulate the breath throughout the day. We create a daily breathing routine much like we create a daily posture routine. Though breathing is typically involuntary, consciously setting out to shape our breathing turns it into a voluntary effort.

Much as we train ourselves to form new habits related to nonviolence, nonstealing, and other aspects of the One Plan, creating a conscious breathing habit requires us to shift unbeneficial behaviors into beneficial ones. Eventually, however, our bodies begin to respond to the consistent shift toward slower, fuller breaths, and breathing becomes an unconscious habit once again. The body's systems then perform optimally: the digestive system becomes less volatile, the nervous system becomes more grounded, the circulatory system becomes more efficient, the immune system becomes more effective, and every other aspect of our physiology comes into a state of balance. Rather than undermining our intention to live a healthier life, our bodies begin to support it.

The Mind: Breath Control Diminishes Suffering

Breath control is unique in the Eightfold Path, in that its basis in the respiratory system requires us to use body's organs to regulate certain vital functions, but the practice itself has a specific effect on the mind. Voluntary use of the breath creates calm, focus, and a sense of grounding—but it also leads to a more spiritually minded awareness. The practice may begin with the body, but its effects have an impact on the mind as well.

Each person has a vital energy force that exists throughout the body. In Chinese traditions, this force is called *chi*. In Indian traditions, it is called *prana*. The word *pranayama* is based on this term, for in creating a conscious breathing practice, we are drawing out (*ayama*) our life force (*prana*). This force is a natural extension of our spirit, and through the use of certain techniques we can harness the force and let it wash over us like an energy shower.

Our life force is affected by our constitution, our lifestyle, our health, and our circumstances. We might experience airiness and excessive movement in the body because our lives are filled with too much of both, or we might experience excessive heat because we are particularly active. We experience stagnation when we eat large amounts of heavy food. But these qualities are not just a reflection of our life circumstances but a reflection of the prana that encapsulates our thoughts. As we learned in Weeks 17–18, each of us has a basic constitution or prakruti. The sensitivities of this constitutional nature are defined by the qualities of our prana. Thus Pitta-like prana can lead to a buildup of heated, irritable thoughts, Kapha-like prana can lead to a buildup of heavy and lethargic thoughts, and Vata-like prana can lead to a buildup of airy, scattered thoughts. Particular breathing practices can manipulate the prana to reverse this airiness, irritation, or stagnation. Once we've altered our flow of prana to attain greater balance in the mind, we are no longer burdened by our egos and no longer experience the turmoil of emotional reactions. We no longer impose our perceptions on our surroundings and perpetuate our own suffering.

The Spirit: Breath Control Creates Balance

When we take command of the breath, we create a shift in body and mind. Breath control makes the body healthier, which allows the mind to move into a state of greater balance and peace. The oxygen we breathe in is converted to a vital force inside us, which then elevates the functions of the mind. The mind takes on an ethereal quality. With a dedicated practice of controlling the breath, we experience a liberation of the spirit that ultimately connects us with all living things. As we work our way into the realm of the spirit, the breath that simply filled our lungs with oxygen begins to lead to more complex practices and experiences. Yogic tradition teaches us that this life force is divided into five forms, with prana being the primary force that moves life forward and the other four vital energies deriving from it. There is *apana,* which facilitates downward movement, such as when we eliminate or a woman gives birth. *Udana* facilitates upward movement and growth, including speech and self-expression. *Samana* is responsible for digestion as well as the absorption and processing of oxygen. And *vyana* facilitates circulation—both of material substances, like food and water, and of thoughts in the mind. In the most evolved breath control practices, we work to manipulate these five pranas within the framework of the body and mind and align them to work in total balance.

Breath control is the first practice on the Eightfold Path that specifically empowers us to move the mind into a new state of being. When the body and mind form a union and this state has been attained, the mind is successfully out of the way so that the spirit may emerge and shine its light on the rest of the world.

The Plan

Your work in breath control will call on you to develop a more beneficial breathing habit throughout the day, starting with a daily practice of breathing exercises much like your daily practice of postures. You may find that you must start off in the realm of the body, or you may already have a breathing practice and will benefit more from exploring the realm of the mind or spirit. But regardless of your experience with this type of practice, you will learn a variety of ways to explore it.

The Realm of the Body

Earlier I explained that we usually take shallow breaths, and taking what we think of as a deep breath is the kind of breathing we're supposed to be doing all the time. Your work in the realm of the body is to explore this deeper breathing through *full breath*. This will become both a habit and a daily practice. This deeper, slower breath uses the full capacity of the lungs, and incorporating it into our daily lives not only leads to greater health and longevity but is the foundation on which you will build up to more developed practices.

WEEK 29, DAY 1: LEARN HOW TO TAKE A FULL BREATH

To breathe a full Yogic breath, fully expand the abdomen as you inhale for several counts and then contract the abdomen as you exhale for twice as many counts.

1. After completing your Yoga posture practice in the morning, lie on your back on the floor with a large book (like a dictionary) nearby.

2. Place the book on your belly. If you breathe a typical, shallow breath, you likely won't see the book move much, if at all. Allow yourself to breathe this way for a few moments.

3. To practice the full breath, inhale through the nose, allowing your abdomen to expand but not to the point of forcing the breath or exaggerating the action. Watch the book rise.

4. Exhale slowly through the nose, as you watch the book lower.

5. Continue this process of watching the book rise and fall with your breath for five to ten minutes. Remember to inhale and exhale slowly. Once you form this habit, this is how you will breathe throughout the day.

WEEK 29, DAYS 2–7: INCORPORATE FULL BREATH INTO THE REST OF YOUR DAY

Full breath is not something to be practiced for a few minutes and then forgotten for the rest of the day. Now that you've learned how to breathe properly, your next step is to begin incorporating this breathing into the rest of your day. It would be nice to tell ourselves, "Okay, breathe fully each and every moment of your day," but as your work with the Presence Practice has likely already taught you, healthy habits must be built over time. To incorporate full breath into your daily life, take the following steps.

- DAY 2: Program your phone, your online calendar, or some other device that you keep with you all the time to go off at about 1 P.M. When the alarm goes off, stop what you are doing and take three to five full breaths. Then resume your activity.

- DAY 3: Follow the same plan as Day 2, but this time set your alarm to remind you to breathe twice during the day—once at noon and once at 6 P.M.

- DAY 4: Set your alarm to remind you to breathe three times during the day—at 10 A.M., at 3 P.M., and at 8 P.M.

- DAY 5: Set your alarm to remind you to breathe four times during the day—at 9 A.M., at noon, at 4 P.M., and at 8 P.M.

- DAY 6: Set your alarm to remind you to breathe five times during the day—at 9 A.M., at 11 A.M., at 2 P.M., at 5 P.M., and at 8 P.M.

- DAY 7: Set your alarm to remind you to breathe six times during the day— at 9 A.M., at 11 A.M., at 1 P.M., at 4 P.M., at 6 P.M., and at 8 P.M.

WEEK 30: CONTINUE BUILDING YOUR FULL BREATH HABIT

Each day this week, practice the same routine as Day 7 of Week 29. This will help you develop the habit of breathing fully all day long, not just when the alarm sounds.

Though developing a full breath habit is a major part of using the breath as a tool on the Yogic path, it is only one part. The other part is deliberately controlling the breath for a specific time each day. These next two weeks of the One Plan will lay the foundation for a breathing practice that will be built over time. The first step in creating this practice is to sit in silence after your posture practice and practice full breath. To do so, follow these steps.

1. Once you have completed your posture practice, take a comfortable cross-legged position on the floor.

   a. Make sure your pelvis is at the same height or higher than your knees, and your spine is perfectly upright.

   b. If your knees are off the ground or your spine is slumped forward, place a stack of blankets, a very firm cushion, a rolled up mat, some thick books, or another firm object under your bum so that your pelvis is higher than your knees. If this is your first time sitting like this and you are new to postures, you will likely need this support.

   c. If you are still slumping forward and feeling intense discomfort, you may sit on the front edge of a chair or stool and conduct this practice with your feet flat on the floor in front of you. Be sure to avoid resting against the back of the chair, though, as keeping an erect spine is an important part of this process.

2. Once you are seated, close your eyes and begin to use full breath.

   a. Inhale until you can't inhale without forcing the breath. Breathing should flow easily.

   b. Exhale, relaxing the chest, then pull the abdomen about halfway in. Don't contract the abdomen tightly.

   c. Inhale and exhale for a longer count as you become more adept.

3. Set a timer and practice for two minutes on Day 1 of Week 31.

4. Incrementally build the time you pursue this practice by one minute each morning for Weeks 31–32. On the fourteenth day you should be breathing for fifteen minutes.

5. Incorporate this routine of sitting and breathing for fifteen minutes after your posture practice on an ongoing basis.

When sitting in silence for these fifteen minutes, you may find that your mind starts to wander or you grow impatient. This is perfectly okay. It's typical for such struggles to take place at the beginning of practice. As you sit, focus your thoughts on your breath as you inhale and then exhale. Simply watch the breath as if you were watching the respiration of animated lungs on a screen. When you realize that your thoughts have strayed from your breath, simply return them to it. This process of focusing your thoughts is great training for steps later in the program.

WEEKS 33–34: CREATE A FULL BREATH PRACTICE AT NIGHT

Returning to the breath after a long and stressful day serves to quiet the mind and ensure a restful night's sleep. Follow the routine from Weeks 31–32, but do so right before bed, or at least within the last hour or two before going to sleep. This is in addition to the morning practices you've already built through Week 32.

WEEKS 35–36: PRACTICE FULL BREATH IN RESPONSE TO ADVERSITY

The purpose of the exercises for Weeks 29–30 was to develop a fuller breathing habit throughout the day. Though the alarms can help you take first steps toward developing this habit, the real work begins when you remind yourself to breathe when faced with stress, tension, conflict, anxiety, or anything else that would typically affect your breathing. Your task for Weeks 35–36, on top of continuing your morning and evening breathing routines, is to use the Presence Practice to remind yourself to take full breaths during times of adversity. At the beginning of your five minutes, ask yourself what you do at such moments—perhaps breathing shallowly, quickly, or not at all. Then, using the following examples as a starting point, ask yourself when you are most likely to do this. Consider one of these moments throughout the five minutes of Presence Practice. You will likely encounter other adverse situations later, which you can add to the list. Do you compromise your breath

- when you have too many things to do at work?

- when your boss gets mad over a mistake you or someone else made?

- when you find out that layoffs are possible?

- when you are late for an appointment?

- when someone cuts you off while driving?

- when you just miss a bus or train?

- when you are running late and can't find a parking space at the store?

- when you don't get your way?

- when you get stuck behind a slow customer in the checkout line at the store?

- when you find out that you didn't get an opportunity you were hoping for?

- when you're nervous about speaking in front of others?

- when someone you live with leaves a mess?

- when your pet or small child has made a mess of your home?

- when you hear one of your children say something rude or unkind?

- when you receive bad news about the health of a loved one?

- when you drop something on the floor and reach to grab it quickly?

- when you observe someone do something you consider disrespectful or shameful?

When you encounter a situation in which you disturb your breath, take three or four full breaths and then continue on with your day.

Practicing full breath throughout the day and as a daily routine will help you find greater balance in your thoughts and lessen the severity of your emotions. When you find that you're falling back into old habits of breathing quickly and shallowly or holding your breath, return to the exercise used in Weeks 29–30 and slowly reestablish your full breath habit. Remember, when you control your breathing, you will control your reactions to people and situations. It is lifesaving.

The Realm of the Mind

Once you have developed a sustainable habit of using full breath throughout the day and you are consistently following a dedicated breathing practice, you are ready to begin shifting your life force in deliberate ways.

We have various types of energy in our bodies and minds. We have warm, masculine energy in our bodies, and we have cool, feminine energy. We have motion, and we have inertia, action and reflection. Polarized attributes are constantly at play in each of us and create energetic disparities. Often those disparities become extreme and cause us to become particularly irritable or lazy, frenetic or tired, manic or depressed. We have an opportunity to create balance between these opposites—to lessen the disparity—by practicing a breathing technique known as *nadi suddhi,* or alternate nostril breathing. Though practicing this method uses full breath, we are now using a technique that specifically brings unity to the opposite qualities of body and mind.

Though you will use the rhythm of full breath throughout, alternate nostril breathing will gradually replace much of the time committed to full breath in your morning routine. To complete one cycle of alternate nostril breath, sit upright and follow these steps:

1. Bring the pointer and middle finger of your right hand to your palm. This will leave your thumb sticking out on one side and the ring and small fingers sticking out on the other.

2. Put the tips of the thumb and ring finger on either side of your nostrils.

3. Close the right nostril with your thumb and inhale a full breath, until the chest has expanded but the inhalation is not forced into the throat.

4. Cover the left nostril with your ring finger and exhale fully through the right nostril, pulling the abdomen about halfway in.

5. Inhale a full breath through your right nostril.

6. Cover your right nostril with your thumb, and exhale a full breath through the left nostril.

7. Repeat. Longer breaths may be built up over time.

The first phase of this part of the program is to replace, over three weeks, the fifteen minutes of full breathing that you've been doing with five minutes of full breath and ten minutes of alternate nostril breathing. Each day, subtract thirty seconds from your full breath practice and add it to your alternate nostril breathing practice. Thus on Day 1, you will practice full breath for fourteen minutes and thirty seconds and alternate nostril breathing for thirty seconds.

On Day 2, practice full breath for fourteen minutes and alternate nostril breathing for one minute. By Day 20, you will be practicing full breath for five minutes and alternate nostril breathing for ten minutes. Repeat this routine on Day 21.

At the beginning of Week 32, you will start adding more alternate nostril breathing to your routine. Add thirty seconds each day, until you have added five minutes. Thus on Day 1, you'll practice full breath for five minutes but alternate nostril breathing for ten minutes and thirty seconds. On Day 2, your alternate nostril breathing will be at eleven minutes. Continue building this way until Day 10, at which point you will be practicing full breath for five minutes and alternate nostril breathing for fifteen minutes. Repeat this routine for Days 11–14.

WEEKS 34–36: EXPERIMENT WITH OTHER BREATHING PRACTICES

Grounding oneself in basic breathing practices, such as full breath and alternate nostril breathing, will take several years of daily practice. It also takes continued daily practice to maintain the mastery over time. However, you may also benefit from exploring methods that affect the quality of your mind. The techniques that follow are designed to cool, heat, or ground the mind and body. For the final three weeks of your breathing practice in the realm of the mind, you are to choose one of the following techniques for each week and commit to practicing it for two to three minutes after you finish your twenty minutes of full breath and alternate nostril breathing.

SHITALI BREATHING: Do you remember trying to fold your tongue into a *U* when you were a kid? Well, little did you know that this trick would be your training for a breathing technique that cools off the body and mind. If you have a propensity to sweat, break out in hives or rashes, or are prone to having many irritable thoughts, then you likely have excess heat in your body. Shitali breathing will help you cool off and find greater comfort throughout the day. Do not practice this technique if you have high blood pressure. To practice shitali breathing, take the following steps:

1. Sit upright and take a couple of full breaths.

2. Fold the tongue into a *U* shape.

3. Inhale through the *U,* using full breath.

4. Exhale through the nose, using full breath.

5. Repeat.

BREATH OF FIRE: This is a popular breathing practice in Yoga studios because, like power Yoga sessions, it creates a lot of heat in the body. This practice is not intended, however, for people who are always on the go and crave lots of activity. Breath of fire is used for those who feel lethargic, stuck, or without enough movement in their lives. Typically, they have excess weight or their body is naturally cooler. Use breath of fire to reverse this stagnant situation. To practice breath of fire, take the following steps:

1. Sit upright and take a couple of full breaths.

2. Begin to force your breath out through your nose, while allowing air to come back in through your nose automatically.

3. Each time you breathe out, forcefully contract your abdomen.

4. Start by exhaling about every second, gradually speeding up your breathing.

5. Toward the end of this round of breathing, begin to slow down your exhalations and finish the round with several regular full breaths.

It is best to watch the video that teaches this method on my website to master the technique.

BELLOWS BREATH: Bellows breath is similar to breath of fire, but rather than forcing air out only through the exhale, both the inhale and the exhale are forceful. Bellows breath is useful for resolving congestion and mucus buildup in the respiratory system, strengthening the immune system, and overcoming sexual debility. To practice bellows breath, take the following steps:

1. Sit upright and take several full breaths.

2. Force out the exhale through your nose, and then inhale through your nose with comparable energy.

3. When you practice bellows breath, the abdomen quickly expands and contracts like a bellows. At no point should you need to strain to maintain the technique.

UJJAYI BREATH: It is common in Yoga studios to place emphasis on using *ujjayi* breath while practicing postures. This is a breathing technique that uses constriction of the throat to retain and manage heat in the body. The word *ujjayi* means "to conquer," and the person who uses this technique will build up movement and rejuvenating energy in the body that will prepare him or her for overcoming obstacles. Use this technique when you feel daunted by a particularly large or cumbersome task. To learn and practice ujjayi breath, take the following steps:

1. Breathe on your hand as if it were a window that you were fogging up. The sound you make represents the constriction of the throat that defines this technique.

2. Practice breathing in this way, but this time through the nose and with the mouth closed.

3. Now inhale while maintaining the same constriction of the throat. In both inhalations and exhalations, you should hear a contained version of the sound you make when you fog a window.

SUN AND MOON BREATHING: If alternate nostril breathing creates balance between the polarized energies in the body, then focusing on one nostril or the other nudges energy in one direction. Sun breathing is used for the same reasons as fire or bellows breath: it creates heat for purification of the body, but in a more gentle way. Moon breathing creates coolness in the body, similar to shitali breathing but with greater emphasis on nurturing and creating calm. To practice sun breathing, take the following steps:

1. Bring the pointer and middle finger of your right hand to your palm as you did for alternate nostril breathing.

2. Bring the tips of the thumb and ring finger to either side of your nostrils.

3. Close the left nostril with your ring finger, and inhale a full breath through the right nostril until the chest has expanded but the inhalation is not forced into the throat.

4. Cover the right nostril with your thumb, and exhale fully through the left nostril while squeezing the stomach about halfway in.

5. Repeat by once again closing the left nostril and breathing in through the right.

Moon breathing is the opposite: you breathe in through the left and out through the right. Both techniques incorporate full breath.

HUMMING BEE BREATH: We often find ourselves in a situation where we want to focus on calming down—especially after experiencing particularly intense emotions. Humming bee breath is a simple exercise for allowing something that has affected us to cease being important. This happens in part because we block out stimulation through humming. To practice humming bee breath, take the following steps:

1. Sit upright and take several full breaths.

2. Close the eyes, and press the ear lobes or some other part of the outer ear cartilage over the ear hole.

3. Inhale a full breath, and as you exhale, make a soft humming sound. Focus entirely on this sound.

4. Repeat this cycle several times, as long as is comfortable for you without straining.

5. When you have finished, open your eyes and resume normal full breath.

How do you know which techniques to use? Use the following guidelines to decide. If you

- feel anxious, scattered, and overwhelmed, and the quiz in Weeks 17–18 revealed a lot of Vata energy, experiment with ujjayi breath, humming bee breath, and further alternate nostril breathing.

- feel hot, irritated, moody, and generally fatigued, and the quiz in Weeks 17–18 revealed a lot of Pitta energy, experiment with shitali, moon breathing, and humming bee breath.

- feel heavy, lethargic, and congested, with an overall feeling of being stuck, and the quiz in Weeks 17–18 revealed a lot of Kapha energy, experiment with breath of fire, bellows breath, sun breathing, and ujjayi breath.

The work in this part of the practice is to tune in to what you're feeling at the beginning of these three weeks and then prescribe a few minutes of these techniques. This type of awareness only comes with being fairly grounded in basic practices. At the end of each week, take stock of how you feel and determine if your breathing practice has had any effect. Continue to experiment with at least one of these practices after your full breath and alternate nostril breathing practices as you move forward.

The Realm of the Spirit

Sometimes students in a Yoga studio are exposed to breath retention and other advanced techniques. We have not engaged these practices in the realm of the body or mind, as we must prepare ourselves for many years before we can safely and beneficially practice more in-depth breathing practices. To benefit from these types of breath control, we must be very grounded in our practice. Below is a sampling of these practices, which can also be found on the One Plan website. To shift the mind in this way so that it will become open to the spirit, however, you must be under the guidance of an experienced teacher. Given the strong impact these techniques have on the body and mind, they cannot be explored without proper hands-on guidance. These techniques include:

- Rolling the Stomach (*nauli kriya*) in standing and sitting forms

- *Uddayana Bandha*

- *Maha Bundha*

Breath control exercises direct the five types of prana in nuanced and deliberate ways. After you have practiced breathing techniques for a number of years, these techniques may be useful in expanding your practice. Another practice you will be able to pursue when you've grounded yourself sufficiently in basic practices is alternate nostril breathing without using your fingers. Once you have prepared yourself over an extensive period of time by using your hands, you will be able to manipulate your inhalations and exhalations through one nostril and then the other using the power of your mind.

Many gurus practice full breath or alternate nostril breathing most of their lives in the body without ever needing to do more than that on their path to self-realization. When you are able to embrace these practices as a natural next step rather than as a way of competing with yourself or others, you will begin your transition into the realm of the spirit.

Emerging as a Masterpiece

Adding breathing practice to your morning routine will provide you with a growing sense of calm throughout your day. Scattered thoughts will become more focused, angry thoughts will become calmer, and lethargic thoughts will become more active. By the end of these eight weeks, you will have developed a discipline for attaining a balanced state that will then help you solidify your commitment to this lifestyle over time.

Putting It Together

If you are pursuing this program entirely in the realm of the body, your routine will be as follows:

- Continue your daily purity practices each morning.

- During the appropriate weeks, practice full breath in response to alarms throughout the day.

- During the appropriate weeks, use the Presence Practice to practice full breath during times of adversity.

- Practice the thirteen-posture sequence.

- Practice full breath after postures.

- Take herbal tea twice a day to continue building strength and cleanliness.

- Practice full breath before going to bed.

And remember . . .

- Continue eating half as much processed food and unhealthy substances as you did prior to the program, avoid eating during the last two hours of the day, and release your sexual essence half of often as you did before Week 7. Avoid accumulating more possessions.

- Continue building your nonviolence, truthfulness, nonstealing, and austerity behaviors to the best of your ability. Continue participating in a physical activity that requires presence of mind at least once every two weeks.

- Eat your lunch in silence at least once a week. Go for a brief walk or jog.

- Commit some time each day to an act of service toward a family member, a friend, a colleague, or someone else who crosses your path.

- Consider fasting for a day every two weeks.

If you are practicing exclusively in the realm of the mind, your daily practice over these eight weeks will look like this:

- Spend ten minutes of your morning repeating the Gayatri Mantra.

- Practice the most beneficial version of the twenty-one-posture sequence for where you are in your body.

- Practice your breathing techniques after postures.

- Read the Yoga Sutras or other spiritual material for five minutes before you go to bed.

And remember . . .

- Continue eating natural foods, refrain from eating in the last five hours of the day and after 7 P.M., and continue to have sex in moderation.

- Continue your nonviolence, truthfulness, nonstealing, austerity, and self-study practices, and avoid sexual thoughts. Continue to let go of attachments to people and situations that you are keeping out of fear.

- Continue to take note of your situational desires and create alternate possibilities for your life. Continue to observe your thoughts in emotionally heightened situations. Continue to practice self-surrender in one area of your life.

- Consider fasting for one day each week.

free from the leash

SENSE CONTROL

IMAGINE YOU ARE A DOG ON A LEASH AND YOUR OWNER TAKES YOU FOR A walk through town. After you find a nice place to do your business, you begin exploring your surroundings. The sidewalk feels hot on your paws, and the sun is warm on your fur. You have light fur, so you can remain in the sun longer than your dark-haired brothers and sisters, who overheat quickly.

As you're walking along, you spot another dog across the way. You leap to get to the dog, for that dog has a bottom that absolutely has to be smelled. As you're about halfway into your leap, the leash snaps you back. Your owner makes you sit down, and he hovers over you saying something in a harsh tone. You're not sure why he's talking to you, for you are, after all, only a dog. You and he continue on along the sidewalk.

A few minutes later, you smell something delightful, and as you continue to walk you're able to identify the source of that smell: another dog's odor. What a delightful discovery. Your tail starts to wag as you strain to get more of the smell, only to be forced back again by your owner. You start to bark, for you must somehow convey to him how important it is that you examine this other dog's offering, especially after you were denied the opportunity for a good bottom-sniff only minutes before. Again, he says something in a harsh tone. Again, you have no idea what it is he's saying. You are, after all, only a dog.

Before you're able to reply, you hear another dog's bark. It must have heard you talking with your owner and had something to say about it! Sure enough, when you follow your ears, you see a dog down the street. Perhaps it was the dog that left that spray on the sidewalk! Perhaps you would be able to compare notes! You bark back and start to pursue your new soul mate, when, once again, your owner pulls on the leash. Again, he says something harsh to you. Though you still don't know what he's saying, the pattern you've sensed is that no matter what you want to do, you won't ever have an opportunity to find your bliss. And your owner will have something angry to say about it, too.

You are, after all, only a dog.

The Things We Allow In

We grow up learning about our environment via our five senses: we see, hear, smell, taste, and touch. All our experiences are somehow related to these mechanisms, such as seeing and hearing a movie or touching or tasting a piece of food. When an object reveals itself to us in some way, our senses take in information. This knowledge then stimulates our brain, and we have thoughts about that stimulation in response.

There are different chains of coffee shops that serve many different kinds of coffee, and they rely heavily on the smell of the coffee wafting out into the surrounding area to entice customers. If we were to walk through an airport that has one of those stores, we might walk past, smell the coffee, and think, "Ooh, coffee. That sounds like a really good idea. I think I'll get myself a cup." We receive stimulation from our sense of smell, have a thought about coffee, and then express a fondness for that coffee before slurping our way through the thing. But what happens after it has been consumed? Aside from getting the shakes from having consumed all of that caffeine, that coffee—that enticing, hot cup of coffee—is gone. Only minutes ago, it held the promise of tremendous happiness and satisfaction, but now it no longer exists. Does this mean that satisfaction no longer exists either? This is the ultimate struggle of the human mind and the recurring theme throughout this program: when we seek to gratify our senses with what we find in the outside world, we rely on the world to make us happy, thus perpetuating our suffering.

But how could this be? Isn't taking something in through the senses and then feeling some way about it just the way life goes? The only true source of happiness is what we find within ourselves, and indulging the senses simply leads to emptiness. As soon as the coffee is gone, or the movie is over, or the comfy chair has been taken away, we are left with yearning for more of it. We experience only loss, emptiness, and lack of fulfillment. In the story about the dog, you may have begun to feel bad for him. At every turn, he saw, smelled, heard, or otherwise sensed something about his surroundings. But each time he sought to pursue something he sensed, he was jerked back and reprimanded. He then felt bad because of his disappointment and his harsh treatment. Though no literal master holds us back when we smell the cup of coffee, following our senses is like being a dog on a leash: we sense something and seek it out because we believe it will bring us gratification, but all we get when we try to attain that gratification is disappointment and a sense of loss.

Until we no longer allow foods, movies, music, fragrances, objects, and the other stimulation we encounter to define the quality of our lives, we are tied to our senses just like a dog is forced to go wherever its owner decides.

A Tape Recording of Life

Though we universally fall prey to our senses, no two people's reactions to stimulation are alike. Someone could smell coffee, grow nauseous, and decide what they really want is a glass of water. One person's idea of an ideal beverage could be the complete opposite of appealing for someone else. But why?

During our time on earth, each of us has formed a collection of *impressions*. When you consider your life experiences to date, you might reflect on how your childhood was filled with happy memories, but your young adulthood was turbulent. The man in front of you in the supermarket checkout, however, might have had to flee his country in the Middle East as a child when it was attacked by a neighboring country, but then settled down in a stable and calming environment during his adolescence. Though you are the same age, your different experiences mean that you have completely different reactions to the same movie about a war set in the Middle East: you find it exciting and great entertainment, while for him it brings back traumatic memories of his childhood. You had different experiences before you saw the movie, which left different impressions on you, which affects how you perceive the world in present day, which then affects your actions and reactions. In this sense, a person's impressions are like a tape recording of everything that has ever happened to him or her. Different experiences lead to different impressions, and different impressions lead to different reactions to sense stimulation.

I recently reflected on the significance of some old impressions during the shooting of an episode of my TV show. Between shots, my client for the episode was talking to the field producer and mentioned the Phil Collins song "In the Air Tonight." Right away, the field producer said, "Oh, god, I *hate* Phil Collins!" Then I chimed in: "I actually have fond memories of Phil Collins's songs. That song reminds me of when I was finishing up at my first boarding school." My client didn't really feel one way or another about Phil Collins or that particular song, and the production assistant—who was in his twenties—didn't even know who Phil Collins was.

This recording of our life experiences exists in our subconscious mind, so though we may not have total recall of a given memory at a given time, hearing a song may trigger a reaction. The Phil Collins song was what it was, but we all tapped into our own subconscious minds when we thought of it. We each had a different tape recording, different memories that the Phil Collins song brought up, and thus a different emotional reaction.

Thus not only do we experience emotional reactions to sense stimulation, but the quality of those reactions is affected by the experiences we have had in life. Having certain impressions can lead to particularly intense emotional reactions ("I really hate it when they show Middle Easterners in such a violent light"), and having intense emotional reactions leads to suffering. When we change the impressions we collect, we can break away from having intense emotional reactions to the world around us; when we no longer have such reactions, we no longer suffer. This promise of no longer suffering as a result of stimulation from the outside world forms the basis of sense control.

Withdrawing the Senses

Patanjali described sense control—also known as *pratyahara*—as withdrawing the senses from the stimulation of the outside world. But how can this happen? Aren't the senses always taking in the outside world? Isn't trying not to see an object that's in front of us the same as trying not to think of a purple elephant when someone says, "purple elephant"? Though an object in front of us may be a form of stimulation, we have the potential to take in the object as information but not react one way or another about it. Rather than saying to ourselves, "Ooh . . . coffee," we're simply registering a smell much like we observe our thoughts during self-study. As the fifth step of the Eightfold Path, the purpose of sense control is to eliminate relying on the outside world for sense gratification and instead to allow our senses to draw upon the perfection of our divine light within.

Sense control is based on the idea that the world around us may be filled with coffee, movies, and many other products and distractions, but within is our spirit—the source of all fulfillment and contentment. In practicing sense control, we flip our senses around as if they were a two-way mirror: after looking through the transparent side to see the impurities of the world around us, we flip it around to reflect the purity inside. When we see this light, we no longer see outside stimulation as the source of happiness, and are therefore no longer taken in by beverages that will never satisfy our caffeine addiction, violent films that will never fulfill our fantasies, and the rest of the outside world that will never help us realize our purpose. In instructing us to control our senses, Patanjali knew how easily our senses could be taken over by the outside world and how overwhelming sensory stimulation could be. He wrote these words over two thousand years ago, before electricity or modern industry was invented, so you can imagine how he might respond to the sensory stimulation of something like Times Square.

Like all practices outlined in this program, sense control manifests in various ways depending on the realm. But the basic purpose is to change the nature of the impressions that we take in through the senses so that we leave a different tape recording on our minds. Rather than feeding our senses with the sights and sounds of violent movies, we feed them images and sounds that are natural and balanced. Rather than chasing the smell of coffee, we purify the air with incense. Through sense control, we purify the impressions we leave on our subconscious mind so that, when we receive stimulation from an image, song, smell, or other aspect of our surroundings, we no longer seek out that stimulation as the basis of our happiness. We no longer suffer in response to what we take in.

Sense Control in the Three Realms

As the fifth aspect of the Eightfold Path, sense control is in a uniquely central position. The practice of postures is primarily physical, preparing the body for higher pursuits of the mind. The practice of breath control utilizes the physical body to affect mental capacity. The practice of sense control, by contrast, makes use of our physical surroundings to subtly shift the mind so it does not react to anything and become disturbed. This practice evolves as we move from the realm of the body into the realm of the mind and onward. Once you begin to practice sense control, it will quickly become apparent how much of life is influenced by your relationship to your surroundings.

The Body: Reduce and Abstain

For thousands of years, people existed in a simple relationship with the world around, working with or on the land to sustain life. The sights taken in came from nature, as did the sounds and smells. The body touched natural material, and food was simple in taste. Now our eyes are bombarded with technology (TV screens, computer screens), our ears take in loud music or the sounds of traffic, we smell poisonous fumes from cars, we constantly touch synthetic materials (fabrics and concrete), and we taste overly stimulating, unnatural flavors.

This sensory overload causes fatigue. Our eyes become tired and dry after staring at a computer screen all day. Our ears start to ring after being subjected to loud music. Eventually, gradually, inevitably, our bodies can't take any more, and they either fight back or shut down. Sleep is the only break we get from the outside world during any given day—and that's only because we're unconscious. Is there any wonder that so many people wake up in the morning wishing they didn't have to get out of bed?

When working with sense control in the realm of the body, the primary goal is to reduce the harmful stimulation we take in and abstain from certain forms of unnatural stimulation completely. We might reduce the amount of TV we watch and instead watch the last ten minutes of a sunset. We might even abstain from certain forms of TV completely, such as a scene that shows two characters fighting to a bloody death. In reducing the stimulation we encounter, we reduce the harmful impressions we leave on our subconscious mind. With fewer harmful impressions, we give our tongues, eyes, ears, noses, and skin an opportunity to recuperate.

The Mind: Shifting the Senses

If our work in the realm of the body is to shift what the senses take in, our work in the realm of the mind is to shift the senses themselves. The senses can be trained to filter out harmful stimulation as we develop greater control over them. A person working in the realm of the body will have to avoid watching a violent program, but a person working in the realm of the mind can watch the program and not be affected by its graphic nature. How might this happen? Earlier we discussed how accumulated impressions inform our reactions to what our senses take in. When we stimulate the senses using specific therapeutic devices, we form impressions that redirect the senses—and therefore the mind—into a higher functioning capacity. The mind becomes naturally attracted to peaceful situations and objects.

This process includes color therapy, sound therapy, aromatherapy, and taste therapy. It even includes surrounding oneself with people who embody the realm of the spirit and share their light with others. On the Yogic path, this is called *satsang*. If someone has a particularly burdened sense of sight (for instance, their eyes are fatigued by spending much of their time staring at a computer screen), they might stare at indigo hues. These hues are associated with the sixth chakra (located between the eyebrows), a center of energy associated with sight. Over time, as the senses are trained to receive beneficial stimulation, they begin withdrawing from the many forms of unbeneficial stimulation around us and are less encumbered by them.

The Spirit: Becoming the Therapy

Imagine if you were suddenly greeted by someone like Gandhi or His Holiness the Dalai Lama. When interacting with them, you would likely feel a sense of calm and peace you don't typically experience, especially when meeting someone new. In speaking with them, your problems might seem smaller. The flurry of events and incidents that have taken over your life might seem less overwhelming.

Once the senses have withdrawn from the world around us, they are left to reflect nothing but this purity within. Here in this purity we find the ultimate practice of sense control, which is to exist within the realm of the spirit while living in the material world. This is where we may provide light and balance to the world around us. It is a light so pure that we become a source of therapy to others.

The Plan

Your work with sense control will develop in subtle ways over time. One day you might be overwhelmed by the stimulation of a crowded city street, and then, after a year of becoming more aware of what your senses take in, you walk down that same street and are able to experience it without losing your sense of balance. This is the nature of shifting from physical practices like postures to mental ones. Through this work, we no longer react as strongly to adverse situations, and as a result we experience more calm in any given moment. And though we may enjoy the tangible rewards of losing weight, resolving illness, or finding other ways to shift our bodies through the physical work, it is in these subtle adjustments of the mind that we find true peace.

The Realm of the Body

Over these eight weeks, your task will be to first abstain from any sense stimulation at all for very short periods of time, and then build a practice of reducing and replacing stimulation over time. The very act of building awareness of what the senses are taking in will help mute your reaction to that stimulation, but the techniques will help relieve your senses of the burden they bear as they're inundated with the modern world on a daily basis.

WEEKS 37–39: BUILD A YONI MUDRA PRACTICE

You may already be familiar with the image of a peaceful yogi sitting in meditation with fingers arranged in a specific way. Usually this arrangement includes the thumb and index fingers touching and the middle, ring, and pinky fingers extended. This arrangement of the fingers is known as a *mudra,* and it is used to stimulate the mind through the power it holds. The mudra just described, known as *gyan* or *chin mudra,* helps develop the intellect and foster happiness. Yogic tradition provides us with various mudras, but for sense control we are going to learn one known as *yoni mudra.*

Yoni mudra prevents the senses from taking in any new information by blocking out all information. This is sort of like imitating the three wise monkeys that see, hear, and speak no evil—but in practicing this mudra we cover all the senses with the fingers. To practice yoni mudra, take the following steps from a seated position.

1. Inhale a full breath into the nose and retain your breath.

2. Pressing gently, cover your ears with your thumbs.

3. Close your eyes and gently place the index fingers over the eyelids.

4. Use your middle fingers to close the nostrils.

5. Place your ring and pinky fingers in front of the mouth, gently touching the lips, which remain slightly open.

6. Remain in this position until you must resume breathing, then exhale. This is one round.

By preventing new sensory stimulation from coming in, you are creating an opportunity to impose silence in the body and from there in the mind. This is a physical way to emulate what will ultimately happen when you withdraw the senses over time.

Your task is to experiment with yoni mudra over the first three weeks devoted to sense control. Do this practice after you have finished your breathing practice; hence you will practice postures, then breath control, then yoni mudra in your morning routine. On Days 1 and 2, practice the above steps as a single round of yoni mudra. Then add a round every two days for the next eighteen days. That is, on Days 1 and 2, practice one round; on Days 3 and 4, practice two rounds, and so on. On Day 20, you will practice ten rounds. Repeat this routine on Day 21 and each day thereafter.

If you find it particularly challenging to remain seated for yoni mudra after sitting through breathing practice, you can lie down for the next practice. If you're struggling to hold your breath, breathe gently through your lips while keeping your fingers in position.

WEEKS 40–44: REDUCE AND REPLACE SENSORY STIMULATION

After you've grounded yourself in a daily yoni mudra practice, your task over the remaining five weeks is to explore reducing and removing sensory stimulation for each sense—one week at a time.

WEEK 40: REDUCE GUSTATORY STIMULATION. Many of us indulge our sense of taste more than any other sense. With so many types of food, alcohol, cigarettes, chewing gum, chewing tobacco, breath mints, and even pen caps, we put many things in our mouths on any given day. On the first day, make a list of all of the artificial tastes and objects you put in your mouth and eliminate a portion of them each day throughout the week. If you want to chew on something, replace these items with fennel seeds, which will also sweeten your breath. In addition, reduce the sauces and seasonings you put on your food, so that whatever you're eating keeps its original taste. Reduce seasonings by half on the first day, and then by half again each day of the week, until by the end of the week you are using a much smaller amount than you usually do. Though it may seem like this makes food boring and even unpalatable, doing so will allow you to tune in to the tastes you do ultimately take in with greater presence and appreciation.

WEEK 41: REDUCE VISUAL STIMULATION. Whether we're inundated with advertisements, addicted to violent movies, or just spacing out in front of the computer screen for hours on end, in the modern world we are vulnerable to all sorts of harmful impressions, which leave our eyes tired and our brains overwhelmed. Many of us are addicted to conflict-driven content, like violent movies and trashy reality TV. Every time we watch two people engage in a knife fight to the death or three spoiled rich kids yell at each other for hogging the Jacuzzi, we're welcoming them into our homes as if they were physically present. This bombards the mind with the visual equivalent of junk food, leaving impressions of pain and turmoil over and over again. For this week, calculate the hours you spend in front of any sort of screen outside of your work, and reduce it by a third. If you watch three hours of TV every night, watch only two. Replace this time with interaction with others, walks, or reading. In addition, experiment at least once this week with using some of your screen time to watch something enriching, like a documentary instead of trashy reality TV or violent thrillers. Continue this new routine moving forward.

WEEK 42: REDUCE AURAL STIMULATION. We spend our days listening to advertisements, songs, talk radio shows, car horns, fire engine sirens, arguments between family members, and many other sounds that leave unnatural impressions on the mind—not to mention leaving the TV on way too loud. This can harm our ears and, in extreme situations, can lead to actual hearing loss. For this week, experiment with a few hours of silence while you're in the car, at home, or in other environments that you would normally fill with sound. If you always leave the radio on as you get ready for work in the morning, listen to it for only three days of the week. If you always have music playing when you drive, listen to music on the way over and drive in silence on the way back. Find at least fifteen minutes of each day this week, and all subsequent weeks, to maintain silence when you otherwise would have filled the air with sounds. In addition, replace some of the music you listen to with gentle classical music or even some *kirtan* chanting (you can find this in the new age section). Listen to this type of music for at least one hour this week and each week moving forward. As you reduce auditory stimulation, you'll not only save your hearing but your mind will start to experience the silence that you've created around you and you will experience greater peace in any given moment.

WEEK 43: REDUCE OLFACTORY STIMULATION. Whether we're seduced by the aroma of coffee or gagging over the emissions of a gas-guzzling SUV, our sense of smell receives all kinds of impure stimulation throughout the day. For this week, try to find places with the most natural setting possible (deep within city parks, hiking trails, wooded areas) to take a break from smelling modern life. Perhaps you can eat your lunch at a picnic table in a park or take a short hike before heading home from work. See if there are simple ways to incorporate more time in nature into your week. Regardless, schedule at least fifteen minutes of each day of this week and all weeks henceforth to give your sense of smell a break from the modern world's many stimuli.

WEEK 44: REDUCE TACTILE STIMULATION. If there was ever an indication of how important a person's sense of touch is, it's what happens when people get home from a long day of grueling work. After they get home, they inevitably plop themselves down on a couch and wrap themselves in whatever blanket-like form of comfort they can find. Here, in this place of comfort, the sense of touch gets indulged. While it might seem like it's completely acceptable to spread out in comfort after a day of hard work, this coziness is like the coffee; both are from the outside world, and neither will lead to contentment. When we rely on couches, pets, children, sex, and collections of tchotchkes that we're constantly arranging and organizing to make ourselves happy, we're only perpetuating our eventual suffering. You began giving yourself a sexual overhaul in Weeks 7–8, and you started to work toward owning fewer things in Weeks 9–10; spend this week relying less on comfy furniture for support, especially after a long day. When you get home, or sometime in the late afternoon or early evening, spend at least fifteen minutes sitting upright, either on the floor in one of the cross-legged positions you learned in Weeks 21–28 or on a chair without using the back. Go about your evening as you normally would (chatting with family members, watching whatever enriching documentary you learned about in Week 41), but do so from an upright position. This will put you in a physical position to breathe better, and you will be relying on yourself for support. This will help you train your mind to look within for a sense of peace.

The extent to which you maintain a routine regarding these reductions of sensory stimulation is up to you, but I recommend that you at least continue to make one change to each of your sensory experiences in Weeks 45–52 and beyond. As you replace more and more of the junk you allow your senses to take in with more enriching forms of stimulation, you will start to crave more fulfilling experiences. Simple moments spent alone will lead to contentment, and experiences shared with others will feel far more fulfilling. If you don't make an effort to change at least a few things, it will be far more difficult to keep shifting into a better space in other aspects of your life.

The Realm of the Mind

In the practice of sense control within the realm of the body, we explored how to physically cut off the senses and reduce the harmful stimulation our senses receive as a whole. When we venture into the realm of the mind, however, we work to reduce the stimulation we experience not by eliminating it from our presence, but by conditioning our senses to no longer receive it as information. This practice is accomplished by filling our senses with stimulation that is therapeutic—we stimulate the senses in a productive and beneficial way. When the senses take in beneficial stimulation, they become more balanced. Balanced senses no longer seek gratification from the outside world; instead they begin to reflect the stimulation that comes from the spirit within. These eight weeks are committed to stimulating the senses in a therapeutic way so that you may curb your mind's need to receive its information from the outside world.

WEEKS 37–41: CREATE A SPACE AND PRACTICE BENEFICIAL STIMULATION

You are likely familiar with the idea of creating a specific space dedicated to practice, for this is similar to visiting a place of congregation for religious observance. Going to a specific place helps set the tone for worship. In a practice of sense control, however, creating a dedicated space can serve a similar but ultimately distinct function. In practicing sense control within the realm of the mind, you are to create a dedicated space either in the corner of a room or within an entire room of your home. Rather than a space of religious significance, it's to be a space of sensory significance. It will contain specific sights, sounds, smells, and other stimuli that will help you begin balancing your senses. Over the first five weeks of sense control practice in this realm, you are to assign a space in which this work will happen and then gradually explore balancing practices for each sense one by one. This practice is to happen in the morning after you have concluded the breathing practices developed in Weeks 29–36.

WEEK 37: BUILD YOUR SPACE AND TRAIN YOUR SENSE OF TASTE. To begin balancing your sense of taste, gargle with some sesame oil or salt water to clean your mouth and eliminate noteworthy tastes. Before beginning your posture practice for the morning, gargle with your chosen substance. After your breathing practice, spend ten minutes observing your sense of taste in silence. Pay attention to whether you can still taste the oil or salt water, or if you can taste anything else that stands out.

In addition, you are to spend Week 37 gathering items that will help you build your space. This space will be where you practice postures, breathing, and concentration in Weeks 45–52. It needs to be an aesthetically simple place, for the intention is to keep the senses from being overstimulated. It will include the following:

- A yantra, mandala, or sample of color (see Week 38).

- A recording of a tamboura, a singing bowl, or chanting of om, or an actual singing bowl (see Week 39).

- Incense of or an oil burner and essential oil of sandalwood, sage, and jasmine (see Week 40).

- If you would like, mala beads or a ring of hessonite garnet (see Week 41).

WEEK 38: TRAIN YOUR SENSE OF SIGHT. Many traditions developed from ancient Indian culture assign therapeutic properties to certain shapes and colors. Yantras and mandalas are visual patterns that are traditionally used for their spiritual significance. When you stare at such a pattern, your sense of sight becomes accustomed to therapeutic images; you will then crave more of these images. Therapeutic qualities are also assigned to certain colors. A cloth, painting, or print of burgundy, amber, white, or silver will promote neutral, beneficial stimulation of the sense of sight. Hang either a yantra, mandala, or swath of color facing you, and having gargled at the beginning of your practice, as in Week 37, stare at your visual stimulation for ten minutes each day this week.

WEEK 39: TRAIN YOUR SENSE OF HEARING. Though silence is always beneficial, there are other sounds that are balancing and can heighten our practice. Sounds that have therapeutic qualities include the tamboura, an instrument that physically resembles the sitar but creates a buzzing sound, singing bowls (different size bowls that create sounds that resonate at particularly therapeutic frequencies), and even chanting of certain mantras, such as om. During the ten minutes you practice sense control in Week 39, play an audio file of someone playing a tamboura, using a singing bowl, or chanting a simple mantra. You can find these sounds on my website. This will fill your hearing with balancing sounds. Add this practice to the gargling and staring practices you have already begun.

WEEK 40: TRAIN YOUR SENSE OF SMELL. Have you ever had essential oils rubbed on you during a massage? The oil has healing properties and therefore enhances the therapeutic value of the massage. But our sense of smell can also be nourished by the use of incense and other fragrant therapeutics, such as essential oils of sandalwood, sage, and jasmine. Instead of rubbing it on yourself, you're going to burn it to purify your olfactory senses. And you'll use it every day. For the ten minutes you practice sense control in Week 40, burn incense or essential oil in an oil burner as you continue with the other practices.

WEEK 41: TRAIN YOUR SENSE OF TOUCH. In the material world, we are predisposed to crave physical contact with objects and people as a way to experience pleasure. But the sense of touch can be utilized to stimulate the mind and positively affect the body as a whole. This can be facilitated by holding therapeutic objects, like gemstones, or objects that promote balance, such as Indian mala beads, or even by using mudras like that described in the practices for the realm of the body. For the ten minutes you practice sense control in Week 41, stimulate your sense of touch in one of these ways: place a ring of hessonite garnet set in gold on your middle finger to quiet the mind, hold mala beads in your hands as you sit, or place your fingers in gyan mudra (index finger and thumb touch with other three fingers extended) with the hands palms up on the knees. Add this practice to those already being explored.

Your task for the remaining three weeks is very simple: incrementally increase the time you sit with these five sense therapeutics in your new space by one minute every two days. At the end of the three weeks, you should be practicing for twenty minutes a day.

The Realm of the Spirit

Until now, you've had a specific corner of a specific room devoted to making therapeutic impressions on your senses—or you may even have an entire room devoted to this. To begin moving into the realm of the spirit, you are to turn your entire living space into a place where everything has a therapeutic quality. There should be no objects that incite attachment or otherwise seduce the senses. This means that there are no televisions or other electronics producing unbeneficial stimulation, nor are there any items devoid of spiritual benefit. When you eat, you are to do so only to sustain life. Therefore, reduce your eating to only once every couple of days so as to lessen the stimulation your sense of taste must respond to.

When you have reached the realm of the spirit in your practice of sense control, you are no longer a slave to your senses. You are no longer on a leash. When you see something disturbing, you respond only in a way that might serve the situation or do not respond at all. But most significantly, your lack of a reaction will teach others how to be peaceful. You are what other people crave as they withdraw from their senses, for when they see, hear, and otherwise receive you as a source of stimulation, you help them balance themselves. Here you become humanity's servant.

Emerging as a Masterpiece

As you continue to add practices to your daily routine, it is increasingly important to remain grounded in your intentions for doing this work on yourself. When you originally came to this practice, you probably didn't expect that watching fewer violent films or TV shows and burning incense would be steps you would take on this path. Given that the practices associated with sense control stretch beyond what you likely perceive as a standard Yoga practice, take some time here to remind yourself of why you sought out this lifestyle. Continue to reflect on what your life was like before you began this journey and how things might continue to change as you grow. If you spend less time indulging your senses, what will happen? How will you feel? What will you set out to do with the time you've created by withdrawing from so much stimulation?

Putting It Together

If you are pursuing this program entirely in the realm of the body, your routine will be as follows:

- Continue your daily purity practices each morning.

- Practice the thirteen-posture sequence.

- Practice full breath after postures.

- Practice yoni mudra after breathing.

- Take herbal tea twice a day to continue building strength and cleanliness.

- Reduce the stimulation you take in for each of the five senses over the five weeks, as outlined in this section.

- Practice full breath before going to bed.

And remember . . .

- Continue eating half as much processed food and unhealthy substances as you did prior to the program, refrain from eating during the last two hours of the day, and release your sexual essence half as often as you did before Week 7. Avoid accumulating possessions, and continue to breathe slower and more fully throughout the day.

- Continue building your nonviolence, truthfulness, nonstealing, and austerity behaviors to the best of your ability. Continue participating in a physical activity that requires presence of mind at least once every two weeks.

- Eat your lunch in silence at least once a week. Go for a brief walk or jog.

- Commit some time each day to an act of service toward a family member, a friend, a colleague, or someone else who crosses your path.

- Consider fasting for one day every two weeks.

If you are practicing exclusively in the realm of the mind, your daily practice over these eight weeks will look like this:

- Spend ten minutes of your morning repeating the Gayatri Mantra.

- Practice the most beneficial version of the twenty-one-posture sequence for where you are in your body.

- Continue with your breathing practice after postures.

- Build a therapeutic space for withdrawing from your senses, and work up to twenty minutes of sense control in your new space.

- Read the Yoga Sutras or other spiritual material for five minutes before you go to bed.

And remember . . .

- Continue eating natural foods, avoid eating in the last five hours of the day and after 7 P.M., and continue to have sex in moderation.

- Continue your nonviolence, truthfulness, nonstealing, austerity, and self-study practices, and avoid sexual thoughts. Continue to let go of attachments to people and situations that you are keeping out of fear.

- Continue to take note of your situational desires and create alternate possibilities for your life, and continue to observe your thoughts in emotionally heightened situations. Continue to practice self-surrender in one area of your life.

- Consider fasting for a day each week.

the river begins

CONCENTRATION

I N THE WINTRY HIMALAYAN REGION OF THE INDIAN STATE OF UTTARAKHAND, there is a glacier that has a terminus in the shape of a cow's mouth. In following this glacier, one comes to a place where it melts into a turbulent river. This river traces its journey from 12,000 feet above sea level down to 10,000, to 8,000, and so on. As neighboring rivers join it, it continues to crash and tumble through a valley toward the south and west.

Here, as the mountains change to plains, the river divides into two paths: it pours into a man-made canal as well as continuing on in its natural form toward the southeast. With this division, each half of the river flows less. The canals further divide and find their way through the countryside. They pass through towns and through cities. They are diminished further by smaller distributaries. Eventually, after many kilometers, the river and its canals merge to form a single river once again.

Merging a Canal

Anyone familiar with Asian geography will recognize the river as the mighty Ganges of the Indian subcontinent. At over 2,500 kilometers in length, it takes many forms, moving through various transitions and obstacles, and yet it always moves forward. Though Hindu tradition assigns tremendous holy significance to its passage and many confluences, here in the One Plan the river may serve as a metaphor for the final components of this program and Patanjali's system as a whole.

The sixth step of the Eightfold Path is concentration, or *dharana*. Here we build on our existing practice of controlling the breath and the senses to focus our thoughts on a single object. We may focus on a physical object, like a candle, or on a mental image, like the body's center of energy. Regardless of the object, when we think of nothing else for seconds, minutes, or even hours at a time, we incite a state of concentration.

Concentration is not easy. The workings of the mind can be compared to a river. In our minds, we rely on the outside world for gratification ("I will be happy when I get what I want") and support ("I will achieve my goals when I receive help"). We even blame the outside world for our imbalance ("I feel bad because people treat me badly"). Because we are the only ones who can achieve our goals, create a sense of contentment, or grow ourselves spiritually, this reliance on the outside world prevents us from finding peace. When we don't, we are as susceptible to the sway of the world as the river is to the surrounding topography.

We start our journey through life as a perfect being unaffected by the struggles of life. Similarly, a glacier is pure in its frozen state, lacking dramatic changes, conflicts, or pollution. When we grow older and our lunch money is stolen, a family member leaves, or other adverse events take place, we are exposed to the suffering of those around us, and we take on this suffering as our own. Similarly, the river melts and flows away from the purity of its original state, experiencing turbulence. More and more challenges present themselves to us, and because we lack a spiritual practice, we take on those influences just like the river takes on tributaries coming from other parts of the mountain. We continue to flow down, down, down, and we experience more and more pain.

When we start our practice, whether we're abstaining from acts of violence, pursuing purification, or otherwise consciously shifting to a spiritual path, the topography begins to level out. Though the river still flows along, it no longer crashes down in an uncontrollable rage. However, practice is difficult to sustain. Many different streams converge and distract the mind from its path. Eventually, though, with the help of posture practices and breath and sense control practices, the river no longer crashes down the mountain but instead finds its way through the valley. The practitioner is ready to begin the work of concentration.

The river, previously so tumultuous, now has some grounding in the topographically subdued plains region of northern India. But just as it is about to venture eastward, the river encounters a large dam and diverges to form the Ganges Canal. Whereas the river was ready to progress unencumbered through the plains, this obstruction ensures that neither the river nor the canal flows with full strength and vitality. Just as the canal must rejoin the river so that it may regain its drive, so too must we train our thoughts to converge on a single point. Though the many forms of stimulation we encounter may distract the mind, through concentration we work to bring the mind back to a single point and allow our spirit to emerge, unburdened by the ego.

A Mental Practice in the Three Realms

Concentration is the gateway to higher practices. It is a mental practice, in that we train ourselves to shift the mind away from whatever may be distracting it—be it a shopping list, a troubling conversation, or fear about getting a job. We might focus our thoughts on the tip of a candle flame and say repeatedly, "Stare at the tip of the flame," but then our thoughts go elsewhere. When this happens, we are able to say to ourselves, "That's a thought unrelated to the tip of the flame. Let me return my thoughts to the flame." Then we return to focusing on the flame. This process of training the mind can then be directly applied to all aspects of this path in the realm of the mind. Just like we say to ourselves, "That's not my object of concentration," we also train our minds when we pursue a mental practice of nonviolence: "I haven't found a job and no one seems to be hiring. That must mean I'll never find a job—oh wait, that is simply my ego telling me that it doesn't have control of the future and is therefore making me fearful of it. Let me return to the task of finding a job." We benefit from practicing concentration because by training our minds we can train our thoughts to let go of the ego.

By now, you have probably noticed that what I call concentration closely resembles what the Western world calls meditation. When you see an image of someone sitting still with eyes closed or focused on an object, you probably think, "Ah, they're meditating." There are many forms of meditation, including those taught by various branches of Buddhism, Transcendental Meditation schools, and Kriya Yoga meditation centers. What all these techniques have in common is that they call on the practitioner to focus the mind on a physical item, an image, numbers, or a mantra. When the mind strays, the practitioner then makes a conscious effort to return to the point or object of focus. Here in the West, the word *meditation* is used to describe the practice that Patanjali calls concentration. The practices for Weeks 45–52 and beyond are similar in methodology to so-called meditation practices in that they call on you to choose an object and then continue to refocus your mind on that object, no matter how often or how far your thoughts may stray.

The Body: Using a Physical Object of Concentration

Just as postures can be explored in all three realms while still benefiting the body, we can practice concentration in the three realms while still benefiting the mind. The most basic form of concentration uses a physical object to focus on. This can be anything in the physical world—the flame of a candle, a coin, or even a black canvas with a little white dot painted in the middle. One can focus on a sound. One can even use the body as an object, focusing on the breath or repeating a mantra out loud.

When we practice concentrating on a physical object, our train of thought may go something like this: "Focus on the candle's flame. Stare at the tip of the flame. That candle looks like a candle that was sold at the gift shop in the town I grew up in. How long has it been since I've been back to that town? At least five years. I guess I haven't been there since Mom and Dad moved to Florida. I hate it there. It's so humid—oh, wait. I'm supposed to be focusing on the candle. Stare at the tip of the flame. Stare at the tip of the—has it really been five years? Oh, wait. Stare at the tip of the flame." And the cycle continues.

There are some sessions of concentration where we manage to focus our thoughts on the object the entire time or nearly the entire time, and then there are times when we can't manage to focus for more than a couple of seconds before the mind goes off on a tangent. The only thing that can help us focus better is to continue doing the practice on a daily basis. We then improve over time.

The Mind: Using a Mental Object of Concentration

Whereas in the realm of the body concentration focuses on something in the physical world, in the realm of the mind it focuses on a product of our thoughts. Whereas we say a mantra out loud in the realm of the body, in the realm of the mind we might say the mantra inwardly. Instead of focusing on a picture, we might create in our minds a picture of a chosen deity, guru, or some other figure of spiritual significance to us.

Another way to create a concentration practice in the realm of the mind is to visualize a center of energy in the body. Yogic tradition teaches us about chakras, primary energy centers located in the body. Just like the Ganges River is the product of confluences of waterways that come together to form a single body of water, numerous energetic conduits in the body come together to form a confluence of energy. Though there are many smaller chakras throughout the body, the seven primary ones run up the spine. The lowest, known as *Muladhara*, is located at a point between the genitalia and the anus; the highest, located on the crown of the head, is known as *Sahasrara*. These seven energy centers provide a structured way to analyze how we relate to our basic needs of survival (food, shelter), desires, achievement, love, communication, intuition, and transcendence to a higher state of being.

Though the chakras may be explored in a variety of different ways—and have been by many scholars—we can also use them as an object of concentration. This practice relates to the realm of the mind because it calls on us to visualize a center of energy that exists energetically but not in the material world.

It is ideal for a practitioner who is just beginning a concentration practice to start with physical objects and later pursue these more subtle practices of the mind.

The Spirit: When the River Flows

Concentration is strictly a practice of the mind. But when we attain a state of complete concentration on an object, all other aspects of the world—especially the mind—fall away. We are not in a bedroom, a cave, or anywhere else. There is nothing but the object in our world. Though we are aware of the object and also aware of ourselves, we no longer see ourselves and the object as separate—we see the object, ourselves, and all other things in the world as a representation of the Spirit. In a state of concentration in the realm of the spirit, we and the object are one.

The Plan

Difficult though it may be to focus the mind on an object of concentration, learning the process is fairly simple and straightforward. For the final eight weeks of the One Plan, you are to create a concentration practice that you will then sustain as you move beyond the structure of this one-year program.

The Realm of the Body

Your concentration practice in the realm of the body will center on an object in the physical world. This might be a candle or a photo of a deity, a sound (like a tamboura recording), your own breath, or your repetition of a mantra. Your task in the first four weeks is to choose an object and incrementally build your practice concentrating on that object over time. Over the last four weeks, you will use an alarm to recall you to the object when your mind has strayed.

Your first step is to choose an object. Consider the following options:

- A COIN OR OTHER SMALL ITEM: Some people respond best to simple objects. Choose a small item like a coin if you enjoy the straightforward nature of such an object.

- A CANDLE: The flame of a candle provides a focused but fluid object of concentration, as its changing shape gives it an appearance of activity. Choose this object if you have a basic lethargy about your practice and would benefit from heat.

- A PICTURE: Some people are stimulated by visual images, and concentrating on a dot on a painting, a picture of a chakra, or even a yantra will draw their focus.

- A SOUND RECORDING: The previous objects require sight. Use a sound recording or another auditory object if you prefer to keep your eyes closed. If you respond well to auditory stimulation and find it easier to focus on sound, listen to a tamboura recording, a singing bowl, or another soothing device without melody.

- YOUR BREATH: If you would like to maintain control of your object of concentration and have an affinity for rhythms, take your inhalation and exhalation as your object. Be sure to inhale and exhale through your nose, exhaling for about twice as long as you inhale.

- SPOKEN MANTRA: You might feel more comfortable controlling your object of concentration but prefer spoken words. Say any of the following words or phrases repeatedly: om (which refers to the divine energy of the Creative Spirit), *om namah shivaya* ("I bow to the inner self"), or *hong saw* ("I am spirit").

- THE SUN: If you are in nature and are able to complete your other practices before the sun rises, try gazing directly at the sunrise during its first thirty minutes. If you like this idea but are not able to make it outside that early, add a session onto your daily routine during the last thirty minutes of the sunset.

- THE MOON: Much like you might do for the sunrise or sunset, use the moon when it is clear outside if you are inclined to practice during the nighttime.

Focus your concentration practice on a physical object if you have never pursued a practice like this and most of your practices in Weeks 1–44 were in the realm of the body. You may benefit from spending your first sessions experimenting with different objects, and then choosing one when you have a sense of which one you favor. Choose the method you best connect with. Whichever object you choose, though, be sure to stick with it. Though it might seem like a challenge, the purpose of this practice is to develop focus on a single object. Therefore, stick with the object you choose for at least a couple of years before trying a new one.

Once you've chosen an object, your practice is to focus your thoughts on it. When your thoughts stray toward what you're going to eat after your practice, what sort of tasks you have to get done that day, or other random things, simply steer them back toward your object. Repeat this process until the designated time has elapsed.

WEEKS 45–48

You are to practice concentration immediately after your posture, breathing, and sense control (yoni mudra) practices in the morning. For the first four weeks of this practice in the realm of the body, incrementally build the amount of time you practice, starting at two minutes on Day 1 and adding one minute every two days (practice for three minutes on Days 3–4, for four minutes on Days 5–6, and so on). By Days 27–28, you will be practicing for fifteen minutes. Continue your practice at this duration.

WEEKS 49–52

At the beginning of a practice like this, it can be very difficult not only to keep returning your mind to the object of concentration, but to even remember that you're there to concentrate. Some people's thoughts stray for the entire time they're sitting trying to concentrate! This is why I recommend that you spend the final four weeks experimenting with an alarm that rings throughout the fifteen minutes.

Given that you're supposed to be focused on your object of concentration, wouldn't it be better to avoid jarring sounds like this? The purpose of this device is to help you when your thoughts stray for minutes at a time. The alarm will jar you out of your thoughts about your upcoming breakfast or your shopping list and remind you to come back to your object.

In Week 49, set the alarm to go off every minute. This can be programmed using a stopwatch or another timepiece. In Week 50, assess whether you're managing to sustain your focus for the full minute or if the alarm is jarring you out of stray thoughts as it's intended to. If you're still focused, program the alarm to go off every two minutes instead. Repeat this assessment in Week 51, increasing the interval to three minutes if appropriate. Do this in Week 52 as well, increasing the interval to five minutes. If, however, your thoughts stray more than every minute, keep the alarm chiming at this interval.

No matter what, always remember that concentration—though basically a simple practice—is one of the hardest things we human beings can do. When

Patanjali defined Yoga as the act of refraining from the suffering of the mind, he drew attention to how powerful the mind is and how much it controls the quality of our lives. If it seems like it is taking forever for you to focus your thoughts for even a minute, don't worry. A struggle like that took place for just about every one of the many millions of people who have tried to practice concentration over the thousands of years that Yoga has been in existence.

In other words, you're in good company. Just keep working at it.

The Realm of the Mind

As concentration is already a practice of the mind, you could sustain your focus on a physical object and still advance into the higher states of meditation and oneness. However, if you have shifted your mind through the various practices outlined in the mental realm of this program and you can sustain your focus on an object for a full fifteen minutes at a time, you may find mental objects of concentration to be more satisfying. Explore your concentration practice in the realm of the mind when you have already sustained a daily practice of concentration on a physical object for a few years or more.

As noted earlier, a concentration practice in the realm of the mind centers on using visualization techniques to create the point of focus. Possible objects of concentration in this realm include the following:

- MANTRA VISUALIZATION: Whereas saying a mantra out loud is a physical object of concentration, saying it to yourself is a mental one. To concentrate on this object, close your eyes and say, "Om, om namah shivaya, hong saw, so hum, sat nam," or another mantra a guru has given you, repeatedly in your head.

- DEITY VISUALIZATION: If you are religious, you can use the image of a deity as your object of concentration, be it a Hindu deity, Christ, Mohammad, Buddha, or another divine presence. To concentrate on this object, close your eyes and picture this presence in front of you.

- CHAKRA VISUALIZATION: If you are particularly sensitive to the nuances of energy in the body, you may benefit from visualizing a chakra. I recommend either the fourth or sixth chakra for this practice. The fourth chakra, *Anahata*, originates in and relates to the heart; as the energy center related to our capacity for love, this chakra will help you see the connectivity among all living beings—the very oneness that you will ultimately attain on this path. The inner guru resides here in Anahata. The sixth chakra, *Ajna,* is located between the eyebrows and is said to be our third eye; it relates to intellect and consciousness, and concentration on this chakra will help you attain a state of more perfect expression and intuition. To concentrate on a chakra, close your eyes and picture a blurred photo of an energetic wheel spinning. When focused on your heart chakra, envision a wheel representing love, compassion, and connection. When focused on the third eye chakra, envision a wheel representing contemplation and perception.

WEEKS 45–48

You are to practice concentration in the morning, immediately after your posture, breathing, and sense control practices. For the first four weeks of this practice, incrementally build the amount of time you practice, starting at fifteen minutes on Day 1 and adding one minute every two days (practice for sixteen minutes on Days 3–4, seventeen minutes on Days 5–6, and so on). By Days 27–28, you will be practicing for twenty-eight minutes. Continue this length of practice over time, or round it up to thirty minutes or more if you like.

WEEKS 49–52

Weeks 49–52 of this practice in the realm of the mind are reminiscent of those in the realm of the body, but the alarm should go off only once during your twenty-eight or thirty minutes. In Week 49, begin by setting the alarm to go off after fifteen minutes. In Week 50, assess if you're managing to sustain your focus for the full fifteen minutes; if so, program the alarm to go off after twenty minutes. In Week 51, increase the time to twenty-five minutes, and for Week 52 and beyond, practice without any alarm at all. Once again, if your thoughts continue to stray before fifteen, twenty, or however many minutes, adjust the alarm accordingly.

The Realm of the Spirit

Practicing concentration for a set period of time each day will open you up to finding greater awareness, focus, and contentment in any given moment. But as we move into the realm of the spirit, we are less concerned with compartmentalizing our practice in a set period of time and instead seek the peace and contentment that comes from living in light throughout the day. Whereas practicing concentration in the realms of the body and mind calls on you to practice as part of a daily routine, practicing concentration in the realm of the spirit demands that you concentrate on every moment of every day. In this sense, all of life is a concentration practice—not just twenty minutes at a time.

To explore concentration in this realm, start working with longer mantras. Committing to memory lengthy mantras, such as Hanuman Chalisa or Guru Gita, is a work of concentration in itself, and reciting one every day is as liberating as it is ambitious. Visit my website to find resources on these texts.

If, after many years of practice, you can stand in Times Square and still focus on your object of concentration, you exist within this realm. When you engage in this lengthier daily practice, you are taking a step toward committing to a state of concentration all the time. Once you have immersed yourself in a lengthy mantra practice, you will benefit from living in a sacred space, like a temple, monastery, or ashram. Being in a space like this will allow you to wholly concentrate through service, devotion to a chosen symbol, or any other aspect of this path. Then, once you have completely immersed yourself in light, you will be able to leave this sacred space and remain in a state of peace anywhere at all. No matter where you are in the world, you'll be able to experience all of it as your object of concentration.

Emerging as a Masterpiece

Here, in the final component of this program, engaging in the full list of practices involves a sizable time commitment. The practices outlined in the realm of the body will take over an hour of your day, and those in the realm of the mind twice that time. Pursuing such an involved lifestyle may seem contrary to an ideal life, given how many obligations we have on any given day. However, making this commitment will not only transform your body and mind and improve your quality of life throughout the day, but it will help you attain a state of peace that few others ever come close to experiencing. When you experience difficulty, be sure to revisit your life. What was your life like before beginning the program? What is it like now? Which reality do you want to experience for yourself?

Putting It Together

If you are pursuing this program entirely in the realm of the body, your routine for these eight weeks and all weeks henceforth will be as follows:

- Practice your daily purity practices each morning.

- Practice the thirteen-posture sequence.

- Practice full breath after postures.

- Practice yoni mudra after breathing.

- Practice concentration after yoni mudra.

- Take herbal tea twice a day to continue building strength and cleanliness.

- Practice full breath before bed.

And remember . . .

- Continue eating half as much processed food and unhealthy substances as you did prior to the program, refrain from eating during the last two hours of the day, and release your sexual essence half as ofen as you did before Week 7. Avoid accumulating more possessions.

- Continue building your nonviolence, truthfulness, nonstealing, and austerity behaviors to the best of your ability. Continue participating in a physical activity that requires presence of mind at least once every two weeks, and incorporate full breath into all moments of your day.

- Eat your lunch in silence at least once a week. Go for a brief walk or jog. Continue to reduce stimulation for each of the five senses.

- Commit some time each day to an act of service toward a family member, a friend, a colleague, or someone else who crosses your path.

- Consider fasting for a day every two weeks.

If you are practicing exclusively in the realm of the mind, your routine over these eight weeks and all weeks henceforth will look like this:

- Spend ten minutes of your morning repeating the Gayatri Mantra.

- Practice the most beneficial version of the twenty-one-posture sequence for where you are in your body.

- Continue with your breathing practice after your posture practice.

- Practice twenty minutes of sense control in your new space.

- Practice twenty-eight or thirty minutes of concentration after your sense control practice.

- Read the Yoga Sutras or other spiritual material for five minutes before you go to bed.

And remember . . .

- Continue eating natural foods, refrain from eating in the last five hours of the day and after 7 P.M., and continue to have sex in moderation.

- Continue your nonviolence, truthfulness, nonstealing, austerity, and self-study practices, and avoid sexual thoughts. Continue to let go of attachments to people and situations that you are keeping out of fear.

- Continue to take note of your situational desires and create alternate possibilities for your life, and continue to observe your thoughts in emotionally heightened situations. Continue to practice self-surrender in one area of your life.

- Consider fasting for one day each week.

to the ocean

MEDITATION

AND SAMADHI

WHEN WE LAST JOINED THE GANGES RIVER, IT HAD JUST UNIFIED itself at its confluence with the Ganges Canal. As the river continues on, it is joined by further tributaries that make its flow more powerful. After a great distance, the river finds its direction. It flows through the calm plains region and past the holy cities of Allahabad and Varanasi. It experiences the momentary distraction of even more tributaries and endures significant pollution, yet still it flows onward.

Eventually, the river empties into the Bay of Bengal. Here you see where the cow's mouth of that glacier so far away ultimately leads, as the river converges with the ocean and becomes one with the world's seas in a continuous exchange of water. What once seemed a separate body of water now becomes whole.

Flowing Beyond Words

In attempting to describe meditation to you, I will never be able to give you the experience itself. Nobody will, for describing something like this has no meaning. And yet, nothing on this earth will ever bring you greater contentment. Like the all-encompassing feeling of love can never be fully described to another, meditation can only be experienced. So why even try to discuss the remaining two steps of Patanjali's Eightfold Path? Rather than teaching you how to do it, my role is to inspire you to seek it out. By pursuing the practices set before you in this book, you will create that experience. This is why we are here. Our purpose on this path is to transcend matter and return to the formless purity we are. Each of us is locked up in a shell—the body—and yet within this shell is a universal, limitless expression of nature. Each of us is here to find this consciousness while in material form.

In reading the culmination of the Ganges River metaphor, I imagine you've already figured out that, once we succeed in focusing our thoughts—merging all the canals and tributaries into a single river—our thoughts begin to flow. This is the next step of Patanjali's system, known as *dhyana*—the Sanskrit word for meditation.

Meditation is the state of being that exists after we succeed in focusing our thoughts wholly on an object of concentration. Concentration is the final act in the three realms, for it can be pursued at a physical or mental realm before becoming reality in the realm of the spirit. But once we attain a state of meditation, we exist entirely in the realm of the spirit, which is a journey unto itself. Complete immersion in the techniques of a committed and successful concentration practice will eventually take us into the realm of the spirit. We will be in meditation and the levels that succeed it. Here, rather than separate and distinct waterways that must be guided to convergence, the water flows on its own accord in unity with the Creative Spirit. There is no longer concentration of thought on an object, but rather absence of thought entirely. It is here that the Spirit is revealed and the ego no longer exists.

I can report on my experience in meditation, and I can write about others who have described their experiences. Meditation has been depicted in poetic ways, in literal ways, and in ethereal ways, but in the end it cannot truly be described but only experienced like love or God itself. You will know when you get there, for it is not of this world. Individuals are all unique manifestations of the Spirit, and they each have their own individual experience when they reach a state of meditation.

But while each person's experience has a slightly different shade, all experiences are born from the same source. I have not included anything beyond concentration in the fifty-two week structure of the One Plan, for the impossibility of describing meditation with words renders it an unattainable step—that is, without a devoted and consistent concentration practice over many years.

When the mind eventually reaches a state of meditation, it loses itself in the Spirit. It may be a long journey, but in letting go of the mind we no longer measure time. The journey is therefore neither long nor short, neither hard nor easy. Different influences might have once been a distraction, but now the mind is in the Spirit and no longer has any thoughts about these stimuli. The presence of the Spirit imparts complete balance, becoming a source of peace for those around us. So too does the river become a source of power for smaller bodies of water.

The Ocean

Imagine if you were to go sailing in the Bay of Bengal, and you put more and more distance between yourself and the shoreline. At some point, you would no longer be in the Bay of Bengal but in the Indian Ocean. If you traveled farther still, you would no longer be in the Indian Ocean. If you bore left, you'd wind up in the Pacific Ocean, and if you bore right, you'd be in the Atlantic. And yet, as you traveled, would you be able to tell from your surroundings what body of water you were in? Would the water of the Indian Ocean be one color, and the water of the Pacific another? Of course not. While you might be able to distinguish one ocean from another on a map, when you're there in your boat with the whales and the sharks, the ocean is just one enormous body of waves.

This is the eighth and final stage of the Eightfold Path. It is not a state of oneness with the Creative Spirit but rather the embodiment of the Creative Spirit. This state is known as *Samadhi*. We experience concentration through a concerted, conscious effort of focusing on an object. When we attain community with the object, our thoughts begin to flow in a state of meditation. But when we allow our minds to get completely out of the way of our state of being—when we no longer commune with either the object or anything else in the physical world, "we," "us," "you," and "me" cease to exist. All that is left is "IT," the one residing within who encompasses the without. It is omnipresent and omnipotent, without form, limit, or name. It is the universe within and without. Devoid of interference from the workings of the mind and the awareness of the ego, there is no more distinction between ourselves and the divine light than there is between one ocean and another. Once we've allowed for the free-flowing thoughts in the river of meditation, we become that which the mind mistakenly thought was separate. The illusion ends and the mind shifts into the present infinite.

I can no more describe the experience of Samadhi than I can describe what it means to experience absence of thought in meditation. Much like meditation, it is experienced as a direct result of an ongoing devotion to our practice. However, Patanjali reports that this state comprises different stages. As we increasingly let go of the material aspect of our time in Samadhi, our consciousness begins to shift in ever more subtle ways. First, we commune with the gross nature of our object as two manifestations of the Spirit. Then, we transcend this state to congregate with the subtleties of our minds and senses. We then transcend this state to no longer congregate with any gross or subtle impressions of our bodies or minds, instead becoming a state of supreme bliss. From here, we climb to other levels, such as the astral level, in which we are no longer limited to the finite reality of our physical form. We then transcend to higher Buddhic and Atmic levels and beyond. Once we are in Samadhi, we are by no means done with our exploration of the universe. We are simply done with the body. Here the real fun begins.

Congregate. Subtle impressions. The astral level. Here, in this final stage of the Eightfold Path, our master Patanjali describes very esoteric truths indeed. As a supremely blissful state, Samadhi is a promise to the most devoted practitioner, but not to be scheduled into a daily, morning routine.

This is the One Plan. This program is devoted to the process of discovering that state of oneness with all of reality. When we reach Samadhi, we experience the source of all life within ourselves. The Spirit embodies light, love, and peace without form or limit. There is no distinction from other living beings, or any object, just as there is no division from one ocean to another. In sharing this aspect of the path with you, I play the role of a person describing a flower to a blind person. The description is useful to them, for they will never see. If they were to suddenly gain sight, however, descriptions of the flower would no longer serve any purpose for them. Similarly, a description of Samadhi will be of use to you until you attain the state for yourself. When you melt into the Creative Spirit, your life experience will be like the eternal beauty of a flower frozen in time.

When we were conceived, we began our journey at the mouth of a sacred cow. At the other end of this path, we become bliss. We become light.

We also become our purpose.

staying the course

WHEN I AM WORKING ONE-ON-ONE WITH CLIENTS, I OFTEN STAY with them for a period of time. Whether they live across the country or a few miles away, I spend several days or a week at their residences as we conduct various therapies and routines. The media always seems fascinated by the fact that, at the end of a day of working with my clients, I find a piece of floor somewhere, sleep, wake up and do my practice, and then work with the client throughout the day. "Weren't there any hotels in the area?" some interviewers ask. "Isn't it weird for you to be staying in a stranger's house like that?" ask others. "Why would you do such a thing?" ask, well, pretty much all of them.

Many clients contact me because they suffer from ailments or conditions that have a debilitating effect on their lives. One person may suffer from chronic fatigue and be incapable of sustaining rigorous physical activity for more than a few minutes without getting tired. Another may feel anxious and stressed about his or her life and suffer from chronic insomnia. Though such illnesses have an overwhelming effect on their lives, my clients are used to taking whatever medications their doctors prescribe and then moving on with their lives exactly as they always did. Sometimes their symptoms become less severe. Sometimes they don't. But the patient rarely resolves the condition.

When I work with clients, I introduce them to the regimen that is reflected in the One Plan. I prescribe therapeutics related to Yoga and Ayurveda, including postures, concentration, herbs, and treatments. Depending on the severity of the condition, this regimen may require a significant investment of time—certainly more time than it takes to pop a pill. But even if they're fatigued or haven't slept well in years, or if they experience discomfort or pain nearly every day, they still struggle to maintain their commitment to this lifestyle.

I stay with my clients for a period of time because creating genuine change requires a shift in all aspects of one's life—and staying with them gives me an opportunity to help them ground themselves in each of those aspects. More importantly, however, even for clients with debilitating illnesses that cause them pain every day, *it's still magnificently hard to remain committed to this path*. I stay overnight with my clients because I want to have every possible opportunity to help them create a shift in their lives.

Thus it is not only understandable but expected that you will struggle to maintain the routine I've laid out for you in the One Plan. Some days, you'll breathe properly and remember not to steal parking spaces, but some days you don't even want to think the words "Downward-Facing Dog." You'll feel absolutely justified in sneaking into a parking spot that should have been someone else's. Some days you may even struggle to remember why peace and purpose are worth pursuing in the first place.

This final part of the book suggests ways to overcome the struggles you'll inevitably encounter as you follow this program. My hope for you is that, even if you have a hard time staying on track, you'll continue to find ways to make your pursuit of this path an important aspect of your life. Below are some situations you may find yourself in after you've begun following the One Plan, and ways you may help yourself stay the course.

I Got Distracted for a Minute . . .

You may have started off strong with the One Plan. You may have scaled back your consumption of problem foods in support of your nonviolence practice, sustained the Presence Practice throughout the two weeks devoted to truthfulness, and even made it all the way through the first ten or twelve weeks of the program. Then, whether it was because you were out of town for the weekend or you got sick with the flu and were in bed for a week, your practice fell by the wayside.

This happens all the time. I've had a consistent practice for many years, and once in a while I miss a day because of something going on in my life. If you find that you've been consistent with the program but get distracted for a week or less, your best move is to simply pick up where you left off.

It's Been Several Weeks Since I Practiced Anything . . .

Sometimes you may get off track for several weeks. This could be because of a vacation, a particularly intense couple of weeks at work, or even just a temporary reluctance to continue. During these weeks, you might have continued with certain aspects of the program while others slipped away.

If this happens to you, you may benefit from rewinding just a bit, perhaps to the last component that you made it through. If you got sidetracked in the middle of Week 9, then begin at Week 7 and work your way back up. If you reestablish your participation at a point you've already worked through, you will have more momentum when you get to the week where you became stuck.

My Life Is All Over the Place, and I Never Have Time for This . . .

Maybe you love the idea of the One Plan, fully embrace the prospect of filling your life with greater peace and joy . . . and feel like you have absolutely no time for it.

Maybe you have kids who are always demanding attention, or you have a work life with a constant barrage of e-mails, or you experience some other daily dose of craziness that takes you away from postures, breathing, and every other discipline in this program. This is, after all, what often happens in modern life. With so many distractions coming at you from all directions, you might feel like your life is one big paradox: the situation that brought you to this program is preventing you from pursuing it.

This is okay. Really, it is. Just as working out for ten minutes a day is better than no minutes a day, practicing even a less intense version of the One Plan is better than not practicing at all. If your life is hectic and crazy to the point of keeping you from participating, scale back exercises to a fraction of the time commitment outlined in the book. Throughout the first twenty weeks of the program, and even in other parts of the program, you are instructed to spend five minutes in the morning with the Presence Practice. Scale this back to two minutes. Instead of gradually building the posture sequences in Weeks 21–28, practice only the sequences outlined in Weeks 21–22 through Week 28. It's far more beneficial to practice a little bit each day than not at all.

I Have Time, but I'm Struggling with the Practices . . .

You may have delved into the practices in this program only to find that you're struggling to get on board with the program itself. Why must you clear out your house? Why must you sit and breathe for fifteen minutes at a time? Why must you use your thumbs and fingers to cover up your face for that weird thing in the sense control section? You might have time to do these things, but you're struggling to be patient with the sessions, you find the variety of tasks overwhelming, or the information is pushing you too far beyond your comfort zone.

Your friends who have kids or a constant barrage of e-mails may benefit from scaling back each component of the program. You, however, may benefit from pursuing a limited aspect of the program to the fullest degree. For example, you might find that you do fine with shifting your behaviors in Weeks 1–20 but don't have the patience to create a morning routine that includes everything outlined in Weeks 21–52. In this case, you might include postures and breathing but hold off on sense control and concentration for now. Then, three or six months after you finish Week 36, perhaps you will be ready to begin incorporating the remaining practices into your daily routine.

I'm Unsure What My Purpose Is in Doing This . . .

You may have the time to commit and the discipline to remain consistent, but you feel somewhat unsure as to why it should be an important part of your life. Perhaps you have a vague sense that a healthier and more balanced lifestyle will be of value, but after six months or a year you are struggling to see why abstaining from sexual release or controlling your senses will add value to your life experience.

This is certainly understandable, as our culture puts a high value on quick fixes and miracle remedies, and going against the grain like this can at times be isolating. If you believe in the value of reforming your life with the Yogic path but struggle to relate to Patanjali's approach, consider repeating Weeks 1–20. The abstentions and observations explored in this first leg of the program are intended to ground us in our practice, which helps us explore our intentions for creating change. By reviewing these practices, you will give yourself an opportunity to reexamine the moment-to-moment nature of your behaviors and actions. This will help you find your purpose. With greater purpose, you will have greater resolve to seek these practices throughout your life.

My Life Is Complicated Right Now, and the Last Thing I Need Is Lots of Things to Remember . . .

You may like the idea of practicing, but your life is filled with a lot of little things that you have to remember, and this scattering of tasks is overwhelming you. If this is the case, you may benefit from focusing on one section of the program for an entire year. In doing so, you will become proficient at that practice and can then naturally move on to another one when your life inspires you to do so.

This approach is best explored through one of the abstentions, as these practices encompass the first step of the Eightfold Path. For example, you may benefit from making a nonviolence practice your focus for much longer than two weeks. Doing so will help you feel the satisfaction of taking steps to improve your life without adding to the burden of an imbalanced situation.

Something Significant Has Happened to Me, and I'm Unsure What to Do Next . . .

We all encounter significant life events, some of them life-affirming (getting married, having a child, moving to a new place), others tragic and painful.

When such an event occurs while you're building this practice, you can lose sight of why such work is important, whether it can benefit you, or, when tragedy strikes, whether or not it even matters whether you grow at all. These points in your life can sidetrack you from the program and disrupt your momentum, and they may cause you to feel distanced from the path.

If this happens to you, but you still feel like you would benefit from some sort of change, simply start the program over again. Even if this life event took place when you were well into the program, starting over has both a practical and a psychological benefit. You can explore again why you're on this path and wipe your mental slate clean. True to the nature of this path, nothing in the past matters. All that matters is the present moment.

I'm Doing Well in My Practice, but What's with All the Timers?

The One Plan is modeled on Patanjali's Eightfold Path, and unless historians haven't been completely truthful with us, they didn't have timers, smartphones, or other devices back then. The One Plan calls for practicing certain exercises for specified periods because this type of precision helps many people remain focused on the path.

But Patanjali didn't say we must practice sense control for twenty minutes a day. He just said to practice. I don't use timers for my own daily practice; I work with postures, breathing, and everything else for as long as I feel I'm supposed to that day. I do so from a place of intuition. If you are grounded in your practice and pursue it every day with dedication and commitment, but you find the time periods laid out in this program to be a distraction, then experiment with letting go of the timers and alarms. Pursue everything for as long as you feel you're supposed to on that particular day. If, however, this lack of precision in your routine causes you to lose commitment, then I strongly urge you to return to using timers until you ground yourself in it once again.

These troubleshooting suggestions are simply ideas of how you may adapt the program to your life, and you are by no means bound to resolve your issues in the way I have suggested. Feel free to mix and match. You may get distracted for several weeks and decide to start the entire program over again because it's the simplest solution. Or you may feel unsure of your purpose and prefer to scale back your time commitment on each task.

No matter how you go about resolving your challenges, the important thing is to remain open to change and allow everything to happen as it needs to. If you fall off the wagon and don't get back on for some time, know that the wagon will still be there when you're ready.

Beyond Week 52

As a fifty-two-week program, the One Plan is designed to provide the grounding you need to sustain this lifestyle over time. If you've done all the work you've been instructed to do, you will likely be enjoying great benefits from the health and calm that was probably eluding you before beginning. By continuing the lifestyle that is laid out for you at the end of Weeks 45–52, you will feel healthier, look healthier, and generally be at peace in your day-to-day life. You will likely have come much closer to realizing the masterpiece within than you ever did in previous chapters of your life.

Given that the One Plan is organized through three realms, it might not surprise you to learn that there are ways to stretch this program out beyond a fifty-two-week structure. In fact, if you really took to these practices, you could keep yourself busy with this book for three, five, or even more years.

How would you do this? The One Plan calls on us to first make a shift in the realm of the body before moving on to the realm of the mind. Thus you may move up from the realm of the body in any given practice as soon as you find comfort in the basic practices. Perhaps you have succeeded in eliminating harmful foods and substances from your diet and consistently refrain from eating for the last couple of hours of the day. This means that you have attained a level of comfort in the physical nonviolence practice and are ready to move up to the mental realm. You would then go through the two-week process of the nonviolence practice for the realm of the mind.

You might be wondering, though, whether you should continue with truthfulness, nonstealing, and every other practice outlined in the program. Just because you're re-exploring Weeks 1–2, does that mean you should re-explore Weeks 3–52 as well? If you have gone through the entire program and you're still craving further growth, you might revisit the program by reflecting on your practice for each component. To do this, go through each of the abstentions and observations that make up part 3 as well as the four remaining practices that make up part 4. Review the practices outlined for each component of the program (the section titled "The Plan") in the realm you pursued in the first fifty-two weeks. Then ask yourself a few questions:

- Do I consistently pursue these tasks, at least six out of every seven days?

- Do the tasks in the next realm seem alarming and daunting, or do they present an intriguing challenge?

- Is this work a nearly constant source of inspiration, or is it filled with setbacks and adversity?

If you practice a given set of tasks consistently, the next realm's tasks intrigue you, and the work you're doing is a source of inspiration, then you will benefit from moving on to the next realm. To determine how your next year of work will be structured, go through each component of the program, answer the above questions, and add an exploration of each practice that you think will benefit you in the next realm. You might have pursued every practice in the realm of the body for the first year, and then decide you'll benefit from exploring nonviolence, nonstealing, purity, self-study, self-surrender, postures, and breathing in the realm of the mind. You would then craft a program that covers the twenty-six weeks of those components.

Or you could just go through the entire fifty-two-week program again, and—to use the above example again—pursue nonviolence in the realm of the mind, repeat truthfulness in the realm of the body, practice nonstealing in the realm of the mind, and so on. No matter how you approach it, though, the incremental nature of adding practices to those you already pursue means that you keep yourself busy with these until you're comfortable in the realm of the mind and ready to explore the many opportunities for fulfillment in the realm of the spirit.

Giving Yourself Life

Giorgio Vasari tells a funny story in his biography of Michelangelo. After Michelangelo completed the *David*, the sculpture was moved to its first home at the entrance of Florence's Palazzo della Signoria. One day, when the scaffolding was still up around the sculpture and Michelangelo was tending to his supplies, he looked up to find Piero Soderini approaching him. As a great admirer of Michelangelo's, Florence's leader was only too pleased to offer a piece of advice: he thought the nose was too big and suggested Michelangelo whittle it down a bit. The young sculptor grabbed his tools and a bit of marble dust, climbed up the scaffolding, and pretended to chisel away at the nose while letting the dust fall to the ground. When he asked Soderini what he thought, the politician replied, "I am far more pleased with it; you have given life to the statue."

Now, this story is likely as apocryphal as the story of young George Washington and his father's cherry tree. But it does provide us with a way to further explore the analogy between the creation of Michelangelo's masterpiece and your pursuit of the One Plan. Michelangelo spent nearly three years working on the *David* before calling it finished. He spent hours upon hours chipping away at it, shaping the nuances and qualities of his work. Anyone coming up to him and deciding in a few seconds that they knew better than he did what the nose should look like would be disregarding the expertise he had developed through lengthy and thorough immersion in his task.

As you pursue the Eightfold Path, you will be amazed at the way you welcome more positive, beneficial people and experiences into it. Perhaps you'll overcome an illness that has plagued you all your life. Perhaps you'll find a career you love. Perhaps you'll see the world not through what you don't have but through what you can share with others. But in pursuing this program, you are also putting yourself in a very small minority of people who have decided to seek their purpose in life and are not just trying to fit themselves into what others perceive as normal. You will likely be the only person you know who spends part of your morning putting clarified butter in your eyes or taking three full breaths when your phone reminds you to. In pursuing the path that Patanjali has laid out for us, you are chipping away at your suffering, and in the process you will become an expert on the nuances and qualities of your work. Someone may come up to you and tell you—because they suffer—that your new lifestyle leaves something to be desired. And that's okay. You are the only one who knows what the nose must be shaped like, so to speak, and in committing yourself to the path of Yoga, Ayurveda, and self-realization, you will realize a light within regardless of what other people say or think. You will have filled that auditorium with love. You, like Michelangelo, will have given life.

Before I set out on this path, I had great commercial success, but I was distracted. I suffered from the burdens of my mind. But this is why I report on Patanjali's work through the One Plan. Whether we find a path like this through a chance encounter with a stranger or we've introduced ourselves to it through a book, the path is one and the same for each of us. It holds the same promise of fulfillment, purpose, and peace.

It is my hope and belief that if you pursue the One Plan, you will find the peace and contentment that eludes so many. You will find the one person you want to be, and the one life that is truly your own. You will set an example for others and find that more and more people will be attracted to the warmth that you give them. As you continue on this journey, you will find that for every ounce of darkness in the world, there are several gallons of light. I look forward to sharing this light with you in this life and the next.

Much love.

eating the ayurveda way

N WEEKS 17–18, WE FOCUSED ON SELF-STUDY AND THE THREE DOSHAS OUT-lined in Ayurvedic tradition. Since this tradition has developed over five thousand years and Ayurvedic doctors study for more than seven years to learn the precepts, it is not a surprise that Ayurveda provides extensive information regarding the best way to eat.

If you consult my website, my mobile apps, and my other outlets, you will find a great deal of information about food, doshas, and how to craft eating habits specific to your body's nature. This overview will provide some guidance when you reform your eating habits in Weeks 1–2, and when you are wondering what should fill up some of the empty space in your refrigerator during Weeks 9–10.

Dosha-Friendly Foods

When we follow the guidelines for eating set out in Weeks 1–2, we are no longer consuming food for pleasure. Instead, we treat food as medicine. Many people suffer from discomfort, imbalance, and even disease when they use food as a way to gratify themselves, but when it's used as medicine, it can help us feel whole, content, and most of all, nourished. This is never more apparent than when you shift your body into a more balanced state by eating appropriately for the doshic imbalances you encounter. In Weeks 17–18, we explored doshas and the imbalances in our bodies. These imbalances can be reversed by eating certain foods.

Eliminate Dryness with a Vata-Balancing Diet

If you have excess Vata energy, you will likely have dry skin, produce a small, hard stool that is difficult to move, have trouble sleeping, and be prone to fidgeting, shaking, or other indications of excessive movement. A Vata-balancing diet requires us to eat foods that nourish the body, moisturize the gastrointestinal tract, and generally build strength and a sense of groundedness. Foods to favor include the following:

FRUITS (SWEET FRUITS IN PARTICULAR): apricots, avocados, bananas, blackberries, cherries, fresh figs, grapefruit, grapes, lemons, mangoes, melons (but not watermelons), nectarines, oranges, papayas, peaches, pineapples, plums, raspberries, strawberries

VEGETABLES (COOKED VEGETABLES IN PARTICULAR): asparagus, beets, carrots, cucumber, garlic, green beans, okra, onion, radishes, sweet potatoes, turnips, zucchini

GRAINS (COOKED GRAINS IN PARTICULAR): oats, wheat, white basmati rice

DAIRY: cheese (in moderation), cow's milk (whole), ghee, yogurt

LEGUMES (IN MODERATION): mung beans, tofu

NUTS AND SEEDS (IN MODERATION)

OILS: almond oil, olive oil, sesame oil

SWEETENERS: natural sweeteners (maple syrup, honey, molasses, jaggery)

SPICES: cardamom, celery seed, cinnamon, cloves, cumin, fennel, garlic, ginger, mustard seed, salt, sesame seed

Reduce Heat with a Pitta-Balancing Diet

If you have excess Pitta energy, you likely suffer from skin irritation, profuse sweating, indigestion, and irritable thoughts. Generally, you have excess heat in your body, and you'll benefit from a diet of foods that reduce heat. This will cause less distress in your digestive tract and allow you to experience greater peace. Foods to favor include the following:

FRUITS (SWEET FRUITS IN PARTICULAR): apples, avocados, fresh figs, grapes (black or red), mangoes, melons, oranges, pears, pineapples, plums, pomegranates, prunes, raisins

VEGETABLES: asparagus, broccoli, Brussels sprouts, cauliflower, cucumber, green beans, green peppers, leafy greens, mushrooms, okra, potatoes, pumpkins, zucchini

GRAINS: barley, oats, wheat, white basmati rice

DAIRY: cow's milk (whole), ghee

LEGUMES: black beans, garbanzo beans, kidney beans, mung beans, tofu

NUTS AND SEEDS: pumpkin seeds, sunflower seeds

OILS: coconut oil, olive oil, sunflower oil

SWEETENERS: jaggery, maple syrup

SPICES: cardamom, cinnamon, coriander, fennel, saffron (it is ideal to reduce your intake of spices when suffering from a Pitta imbalance)

Reduce Moisture with a Kapha-Balancing Diet

If you have excess Kapha energy, you likely suffer from respiratory congestion, asthma, and overweight or obesity, and feel lethargic and stuck. Excessive Kapha energy leads to a buildup of moisture, such as congestion in the respiratory system. When you balance Kapha energy through an appropriate diet, you will reverse heaviness in the body. Foods to favor include the following:

FRUITS: apples, apricots, blackberries, cherries, dried cranberries, dry figs, mangos, peaches, pears, persimmons, pomegranates, prunes, raisins

VEGETABLES: asparagus, beets, broccoli, Brussels sprouts, carrots, cauliflower, eggplant, garlic, leafy greens, mushrooms, okra, onions, peas, peppers, potatoes, radishes, spinach, sprouts

GRAINS: barley, corn, millet

DAIRY: ghee, goat's milk (in moderation)

LEGUMES: garbanzo beans, green lentils, red lentils

NUTS AND SEEDS (IN MODERATION): pumpkin seeds, sunflower seeds

OILS: corn oil, mustard oil

SWEETENERS: raw honey

SPICES: black pepper, ginger, turmeric, and all other spices except salt

Ayurvedic Food Preparation

Whether you have a specific doshic imbalance you'd like to correct or you want to eat meals based on Ayurvedic practices for the sake of improving your health, you will benefit from preparing and consuming simple meals that provide basic sustenance for your body. Such meals consist of several vegetables cooked with some basic spices, white basmati rice, and if appropriate for your constitution and the time of day, some legumes. If you are seeking to balance a particular dosha, favor foods for balancing that dosha. If you are interested in having a generally nourishing meal, select foods from each of the three doshic guidelines. For example, prepare carrots (Vata) and cauliflower (Kapha) with black pepper (Kapha), cumin (Vata), and coriander (Pitta). Serve this with coconut oil (Pitta) and white basmati rice (Pitta and Vata). Take the following steps to prepare a basic dish of vegetables:

1. If you are preparing your meal with seeds (cumin, fennel, mustard), put a small amount of oil in a wok over a medium heat. Add the seeds after the oil has heated for a minute or so. When the seeds pop, proceed to step 2. If you are only using powder, skip right to step 2.

2. Add diced vegetables to the wok with a small amount of water so that the vegetables will be steamed but not submerged. Add the powdered spices and stir.

3. Allow the vegetables to steam until the water has burned off, stirring occasionally. Immediately remove from heat.

4. Melt ghee or pour oil over the vegetables and stir.

5. Serve with white basmati rice, and if appropriate for the time of day and your body type, a dish of lentils or another type of legume.

appendix b

the bigger
picture

THE ANCIENT SAGES OF INDIA EXPLAIN HUMANITY'S STRUGGLE WITH
health and spiritual well-being by reference to a cyclical model of
change. Humanity cycles through a series of four eras, which vary
from the most material to the most balanced and spiritual. Each era, known
as a *yuga*, lasts thousands of years. We are now in Kali Yuga, the densest, most
material period, which accounts for our suffering.

The sages developed the system of Yoga over the course of millennia. The
long history of Indian philosophy that can be traced in its spiritual works, especially the Vedas, the Upanishads, and the Bhagavad Gita, comes to fruition in
the Yoga Sutras. Though Yoga existed as a concept and a lifestyle for centuries
beforehand, the Yoga Sutras accomplished for this system what Newton's Prin-
cipia did for science. Though the Eightfold Path that is featured in the One Plan
comes from the Yoga Sutras, it is only one part of the Sutras' 196 aphorisms. Just
as modern-day books are divided into chapters, the Yoga Sutras are divided into
four sections called *padas*. The first pada provides a definition of Yoga (*Chitta
vritti nirodhah*, or "Yoga is the practice of removing afflictions of the mind.")
and shows how mental suffering plays a role in our lives. The second pada outlines the practical aspects of working toward that higher state (including the
beginning of the Eightfold Path). The third pada continues the explanation of
the Eightfold Path and outlines what we accomplish in the state of Samadhi.

Finally, the fourth pada shows how the spiritual forces at play in the universe affect our existence. Much of this information might seem esoteric to modern readers, but it is presented with usability in mind.

Ultimately, when humanity reaches the highest yuga many millennia from now, we will live and coexist in perfection without the struggle and pain that comes from conflict and disease. When the sages intuited the Yogic tradition through their community with the Creative Spirit, they intended to provide tools for achieving this state despite our predisposition to materialism. Your best resource for discovering the divine light within yourself is the Sutras themselves. Many books provide translations of the aphorisms along with helpful commentary. I encourage you to spend time with this information to help yourself on this journey—and to help humanity as a whole.